Maternal–Newborn Home Care Manual

Maternal–Newborn Home Care Manual

Mary Ann Chestnut, RN

President, Citadel MCH, Inc.
Narberth, Pennsylvania

Lippincott
Philadelphia • New York

Acquisitions Editor: Jennifer E. Brogan
Coordinating Editorial Assistant: Susan V. Barta
Production Editor: Virginia Barishek
Production Manager: Helen Ewan
Production Service: Berliner Inc.
Printer/Binder: Victor Graphics
Cover Designer: Joan Wendt
Cover Printer: Lehigh Press

9 8 7 6 5 4 3 2 1

Library of Congress Cataloging-in-Publication Data
Chestnut, Mary Ann
Maternal-newborn home care manual / Mary Ann Chestnut.
p. cm.
Includes bibliographical references and index.
ISBN 0-397-55474-5
1. Maternity nursing—Handbooks, manuals, etc. 2. Infants (Newborn)—Home care—Handbooks, manuals, etc. 3. Perinatology—Handbooks, manuals, etc. I. Title.
[DNLM: 1. Postnatal Care—methods. 2. Neonatal Nursing—methods. 3. Home Care Services—standards. WY 157.3 C525m 1997]
RG951.C443 1997
610.73'62—dc21
DNLM/DLC
for Library of Congress 97-25845
CIP

Care has been taken to confirm the accuracy of the information presented and to describe generally accepted practices. However, the authors, editors, and publisher are not responsible for errors or omissions or for any consequences from application of the information in this book and make no warranty, express or implied, with respect to the contents of the publication.

The authors, editors and publisher have exerted every effort to ensure that drug selection and dosage set forth in this text are in accordance with current recommendations and practice at the time of publication. However, in view of ongoing research, changes in government regulations, and the constant flow of information relating to drug therapy and drug reactions, the reader is urged to check the package insert for each drug for any change in indications and dosages and for added warnings and precautions. This is particularly important when the recommended agent is a new or infrequently employed drug.

Some drugs and medical devices presented in this publication have Food and Drug Administration (FDA) clearance for limited use in restricted research settings. It is the responsibility of the health care provider to ascertain the FDA status of each drug or device planned for use in their clinical practice.

This book is dedicated to Albert Pizzica, DO,
for his deep commitment to the development of home visiting services and
to the women and infants of North Philadelphia, and for his commitment and his
faith through the implementation of this program.

Thank you for your inspiration and resolve in spite of all the incredible odds.

Preface

The *Maternal–Newborn Home Care Manual* is the culmination of 16 years of work in maternal–child home health care. The program evolved from one developed in the early 1980s to address the needs of postpartum women who chose to leave the hospital with their newborns 24 to 48 hours after delivery. What was once defined as early discharge, however, has now become the accepted standard of practice regarding postdelivery length of hospital stay. The need to provide at least one home visit to all newborns and their mothers has been heightened as a result of the reduced lengths of hospital stay in the 1990s. The trend will surely continue into the 21st century as a result of cost containment practices.

For this reason, persons working in the field of maternal–child health must integrate home visiting into the postpartum plan for all new mothers and infants. Some areas in the United States have created legislation that actually mandates a home visit to postpartum families. Most research done on the subject of early discharge indicates that with appropriate follow-up, the practice is safe and may reduce the incidence of nosocomial infection.

The key is appropriate follow-up. Many conditions associated with maternal and infant morbidity do not present until 3 to 10 days after delivery. Some of these problems include uterine infections, retained placental fragments, and wound infections (in the mother). Problems that most frequently appear in newborns after 48 hours include jaundice, aspiration pneumonia, and infections on the skin and in the cord. In addition to maternal and newborn medical assessment, the home visit provides an opportunity to offer education in a more relaxed atmosphere after the primary stress of labor and delivery has ended.

Chapter 1 of *Maternal–Newborn Home Care Manual* contains personnel policies that are oriented to nurses making postpartum newborn visits. This section will be useful both to administrators for recruitment, orientation, and evaluation, and to nurses providing direct care in the home as a standard of practice. This section is also necessary to any maternal–child service seeking Medicare certification or accreditation by the Joint Commission on the Accreditation of Healthcare Organizations (JCAHO) as a home health agency.

Home health agencies are not the only providers of this service. Often hospitals, birthing centers, insurance organizations, physicians, nurse–midwives, and grant-funded community service programs will employ nurses to provide a postpartum–newborn visit to their clients. This manual will be a helpful tool to anyone attempting to apply and implement quality standards of care in maternal–child home visiting.

Chapter 2 provides standards for the psychosocial and physical risk assessment of both mother and newborn. Included are definitions that will help the nurse objectively define psychosocial risk factors. The standards for physical assessment are very comprehensive and include findings considered to be within normal limits, deviations, and their assessment, along with actions to take when deviations are noted. Nurses will find this section to be a helpful tool to carry in the field for easy reference.

Chapter 3 addresses invasive procedures that may be required at the postpartum–newborn home visit. During the routine postpartum–newborn home visit, the nurse often may perform invasive procedures to obtain newborn blood specimens for metabolic screening or bilirubin. Mothers or infants could also need to complete a course of antibiotic therapy in the home. Obstetrical care providers may request that the nurse also obtain blood specimens to evaluate the resolution of a problem with the mother. Administrators must be assured that persons performing these procedures are competent and practice according to a prescribed standard. Nurses must have access to adequate orientation and a standard procedure.

Chapter 4 provides standards that can be applied to a High-Risk Newborn Home Care Program. A federal task force, convened to study and make recommendations on the content of prenatal care, found in 1989 that a series of regularly scheduled home visits to infants at risk throughout their first year of life could significantly reduce infant morbidity and mortality in that population. The program described here was implemented as a 2-year pilot study. Initial results of the study have yielded significantly fewer hospitalizations and emergency room visits and a higher incidence of adequate immunizations among the infants seen for the first year, compared with those in another group with the same risk categories who were not seen beyond the postpartum period. Although providers may need to search for them, the resources are available for funding to provide continued home visiting services to infants at risk. Many insurers who provide coverage in areas of higher-than-average infant mortality have access to funding for organized preventive home visiting services. Those interested in offering this program may additionally find funding resources through their local Department of Health, their state Department of Health, and the Federal Department of Health and Human Services in Rockville, Maryland (Health and Human Services, 5600 Fishers Lane, Rockville, Maryland 20857). When inquiring, always ask for the Division of Maternal–Child Health. Admission to the High-Risk Newborn program is determined at the first postpartum-newborn visit that hopefully all families receive regardless of risks. Based upon admission criteria described in this chapter, mothers and infants determined to be at risk are admitted to the program and receive a series of visits. The content and timing of the visits along with health outcome indicators helpful to the evaluation of the program's effectiveness are included. Tools to assist in data collection for quality assurance purposes are included in Section 2 of the Appendix.

Chapter 5 contains specific protocols used in postpartum newborn home visiting. Included are protocols related to the newborn such as phototherapy, apnea monitoring, diarrhea, neonatal antibiotic therapy, and neonatal abstinence. Maternal protocols include staple removal, wound dehiscence, and bereavement. Protocols that apply to mother, newborn, and nurse include limiting infections in the home and body fluid precautions are presented.

Chapter 6 presents educational material that can be copied and shared with the family as part of the home visit. Families will find it helpful to have this material left with them by the nurse. The Appendix provides the user with the necessary clinical forms for both the initial postpartum-newborn home visit and risk assessment along with follow-up visits for newborns admitted to high-risk infant follow-up. There are also useful tools to assist in data collection and evaluation, a list of common abbreviations, a glossary, and a bibliography to help the home health agency build its own library of resources.

Mary Ann Chestnut, RN

Acknowledgments

As a nurse working in the field of maternal–child health since 1982, I have had the privilege of working with many individuals who contributed to my knowledge and inspired me to write and publish this manuscript. I would like to thank and acknowledge those who have so willingly contributed this support.

- *The staff of Booth Maternity Center, Philadelphia, Pennsylvania, who are too numerous to list here.*

- *The staff at Family Help, Inc., including:*
  Ellen Craighead, RN, BSN
  Marilyn Kerr, RN, BSN
  Bonnie Charleston
  Anne Ravdin, RN, BSN
  Ann Galanter, RN, BSN
  Joanne Fischer, MSW
  Laurie Reardon, RN, BSN
  Barbara Tinus, RN, BSN
  Gail Pierson, RN, PNP
  Barbara Krinsky, RN, BSN
  Millie Boettcher, RN, MSN
  Patricia Larsen, RN, MSN, CNM
  Debbie Westcott, RN, BSN
  Judy Woomer, CHHA
  and all the other staff who made Family Help a reality

- *The staff at Citadel MCH Services*
  Sonya Newell Wilson, RN
  Kathleen Whalen, RN
  Jacqueline Williams, RN, BSN
  Vicki Newell
  Carol Hallenback, RN, BSN
  Judy Podosky, RNC
  Ann Galanter, RN, BS
  Norma Cintron, RN

- *Also a joint acknowledgment must be made to those who served on The Professional Advisory Committees of Family Help, Inc. (1985–1990) and/or The Professional Advisory Committees of Citadel MCH Services, Inc. (1991–1995):*
  Paul Branca, MD
  Ronald Bolognese, MD
  Judy Bernbaum, MD
  Evelyn Bouden, MD
  Carl Bailey
  Jannie L. Blackwell
  Roberta Capewell, RN, MSN, PNP
  Julia Clarke, RN, CNM, MSN
  Jane Eleey, MSW
  Jeffrey Gerdes, MD
  Page Talbott Gould, PhD
  Howard Grant, MD, JD
  Robert Holmes, MD
  Susan Hutchinson, RNC, MSN
  Mark A. Kalchbrenner, DO
  Rich Kaplan, MD
  June Kinney, PhD
  Rose Kinney, RN, BSN
  Judith McCoyd, ACSW, LSW
  Carol L. Natter, PT
  Lucille Pema, RN, BSN
  Albert Pizzica, DO
  Barbara Ritchey, ACSW, LSW
  Jeffrey Rothirtan, EdD:, PT
  Barbara Schraeder, RN, PhD
  Robert Stavis, PhD, MD
  Patricia Thiebault, RD
  Barbara Wesley, MD, MPH
  Robert S. Wimmer, MD
  Mary Wright, MOT
  Susan Yates, CNM, MSN

- *I also want to thank Scott Bucher, RN and Mylo Woodward, RN of the Pennsylvania Department of Health, Maternal–Child Division, and Frank Heron of the U.S. Department of Health and Human Services for their support and assistance throughout the years.*

Contents

CHAPTER 4

Standard Program for High-Risk Newborn Home Visiting Follow-Up 47

CHAPTER 5

Specific Protocols Used in Maternal–Newborn Follow-Up 59

CHAPTER 6

Family Education Materials 95

CHAPTER 1

Personnel Policies and Procedures

This chapter covers the personnel policies and procedures relative to nursing performance when making postpartum nursing home visits. Administrative persons will find these helpful for job description purposes. All nurses either supervising or providing direct care should be provided with a copy of this section during orientation in order to understand performance requirements adequately. In addition, these standards should be used as a component of concurrent and retrospective audits for quality of services rendered. These standards will also provide a means to assess comprehensive nursing practice as part of the evaluation process for nurses working within the program.

STANDARD NURSING PRACTICE

PURPOSE: These guidelines are designed to apply uniform quality standards in professional nursing practice related to the postpartum visit within the family-centered maternity care program.

RATIONALE: Guidelines are provided for the professional employee for expected standards of practice within the family-centered care program.

CONTENT: The duties and responsibilities of the nurse in the family-centered care program are described below.

1. Receives and records the clinical assignment from the supervisor.
2. Verifies the time of the scheduled visit with the client before arrival.
3. Establishes a client relationship using the "helping relationship" (orientation, working, and termination stages; see Box 1-1).
4. Reviews Terms and Conditions of Services, including requirements for third-party reimbursement, with the client before beginning work.
5. Explains all procedures and rationales to the client before performance.
6. Reviews Patient Rights and Responsibilities as determined by PAHHA Code of Ethics for Home Care.
7. Assesses maternal needs, reinforcing the following items on Postpartum Assessment Tool: breast milk and care, episiotomy, lochia, fundus, voiding, bowel pattern, temperature, pulse, blood pressure, Homans's sign, varicosities, edema, vitamins, iron, fluid balance, nutrition, emotional status, and client's knowledge of infant care.
8. Provides primary instruction or reinforces individualized postpartum teaching according to the type of delivery and the condition of mother, covering rest, activity, diet, elimination, vaginal discharge, sexual activity, maternal activity levels, hygiene, stitches, hemorrhoids, exercise, wound care, breastfeeding, care of breasts and nipples, and breast pumping.

BOX 1-1: THE HELPING RELATIONSHIP

Orientation Phase: The client will know the nurse by name and accurately describe the roles of the participants in the relationship. The client and nurse will establish an agreement regarding:

- Goals of the relationship
- Location, frequency, and length of contact

Working Phase: The nurse and client work together to meet the client's goals. The client actively participates, cooperating in activities to reach those goals. The client can express his or her feelings and concerns to the nurse.

Termination: The client participates in identifying progress toward or accomplishment of goals. The client verbalizes feelings about the termination of the relationship.

9. Reviews normal newborn behavior (types of crying, sleeping patterns, stimulation, and bonding).

10. Discusses self-care measures, employing the concepts of active decision making by the client in relation to self-care needs.

11. Discusses a preventive approach to postpartum depression, stressing key causative factors and troubleshooting methods.

12. Explains metabolic screening testing; verifies if this testing has been done; and assesses the need for repeat testing according to physician instructions for follow-up. Resolves any questions with the baby's primary physician. Obtains a metabolic screening if indicated.

13. Evaluates for the need of Home Health Aide services or evaluates the services if they are already being used.

14. Reviews community resources available to the family (insurance coverage, health clinics, breastfeeding groups, parenting groups, etc.).

15. Provides preventive health teaching concerning breast self-examination; the effects of smoking, drugs, diet, and caffeine; infant immunizations; the need for physical examinations; signs and symptoms of illness in the family and baby; and resuscitative and emergency procedures for infants.

16. Performs assessment of newborn, checking appearance, skin color, heart rate and sounds, temperature, respiratory rate and character, neurologic status, muscle tone, abdomen, neck, extremities, femoral pulse, genitalia, history of voiding and bowel movement, condition of cord, condition of circumcision, nutritional history from birth, and nutrition.

17. Provides instruction in newborn care, reinforcing the following items on the Newborn Assessment Tool: bathing, cord care, diapering and dressing, diaper rash, circumcision care, fresh air, stuffy nose, sleeping, visiting, immunizations, medications, books available, cool mist, temperature-taking techniques, ipecac, meeting the infant's physical and emotional needs, and problems that require special attention.

18. Reviews the patient education materials.

POSTPARTUM ASSESSMENT

POLICY: A postpartum assessment will be performed on all clients referred to the postpartum program.

PURPOSE: The postpartum assessment is conducted to provide nursing assessment for mothers and infants in early-discharge maternity programs.

PROCEDURE: The procedures to be used for conducting the postpartum assessment are described below.

1. The hospital will assure that all women receive access to home visiting nurse services following discharge.

2. The agency or nurse will contact the mother after the referral is received.

3. A visit will be scheduled according to the plan of care.

4. If the nurse is unable to schedule a visit, the nurse will contact the agency with the problem, within the first 24 hours after discharge. The agency will notify the hospital physician and insurer (if required).

5. If the mother is a "no-show" when the nurse arrives for the visit, the nurse will contact the agency with a report on the status of the visit and will continue to attempt to see the mother and the baby based upon additional information the agency, hospital nurse, or insurer are able to provide.

6. The nurse will obtain a signed consent for both the mother and the baby as required.

7. The nurse will perform a physical assessment of the mother.

8. The nurse will perform a physical assessment of the infant.

9. The nurse will perform a risk assessment and determine whether there are additional problems requiring additional home care or follow-up by the physician.

10. The nurse will complete the assessment form for both the mother and baby, clearly noting the mother's insurance number and type, date of birth, WIC appointment, baby's pediatrician, date and time of follow-up appointment, and all other required information.

11. The nurse will ask the mother which county office she uses and will report this information to the agency, including the name of the mother's caseworker. The nurse may also assist in ensuring infant coverage.

12. The nurse will call the county office from the patient's home to notify the county office/caseworker of the birth of the baby and will schedule an appointment to get the baby an insurance card if the mother or infant are uninsured. (Outreach agencies can complete enrollments.)

13. The nurse will review emergency numbers and safety measures with the mother.

14. The nurse will make referrals to other agencies as needed.

15. The nurse will have the mother sign a time log for both herself and her baby.

16. The nurse will notify the agency when the assessment has been completed and will report whether or not the patient will be referred into the home care program.

17. The nurse will return the completed assessments, consent forms, and time logs to the agency.

CHAPTER 2

Standards for Psychosocial and Physical Risk Assessment

DIRECTIONS FOR USE OF THE POSTPARTUM/INFANT UNIVERSAL HOME RISK ASSESSMENT

1. The Postpartum/Infant Universal Home Risk Assessment Procedure includes the following:
   a. Directions for use
   b. The Postpartum/Infant Home Risk Assessment Tool
   c. Postpartum/Infant Risk Assessment Standards
2. A referral form should be completed by the source making the referral to the home health agency. Referrals for initial visits can be made by the client's physician, nurse practitioner, nurse, social worker, the client herself, outreach, or other significant person involved in the client's care.
3. The agency, provider, and insurers will make all attempts to determine whether the mother or the newborn has had previous home care services in this pregnancy to assure appropriate coordination of care, access to medical history, and referral to the previous provider if appropriate.
4. The parent or guardian will be advised in advance of client rights in compliance with federal Medicare requirements.
5. All Plans of Care will be supervised by a physician in compliance with Medicare standards.
6. It is recommended that all newborn infants and postpartum women be afforded access to the Universal Home Risk Assessment, especially those at or below the poverty level, to determine the following:
   a. If there are risk factors that were not obvious during the prenatal period.
   b. If there are any plans for community services.
   c. If there is an ongoing need for home care services.

7. Based on the findings of this assessment, clients may be discharged from home care to their primary care provider or admitted to home care for follow-up based on short-term medical needs of the mother or infant. These areas are those in which the agency anticipates resolution of home care involvement within the first 62 days after delivery.

8. Guidelines by risk category
   a. Initial assessment: All women and children will receive an initial home visit for physical and psychosocial assessment and determination of level of risk.
   b. Initial risk-specific home care
      1) Increased risk: All women and children determined to have one or more level 1 risk factors are eligible for one to three visits per month for 62 days, depending on individual need and per the physician's Plan of Care.
      2) Moderate risk: All women and children determined to have one or more level 2 risk factors are eligible for one to three visits per week for 62 days, depending on individual need and per the physician's Plan of Care.
      3) Maximal risk: All women and children determined to have one or more level 3 risk factors are eligible for four to seven visits per week for 62 days, depending on individual need and per the physician's Plan of Care.
   c. Ongoing risk-specific home care: The risk status of all women and children will be reassessed every 62 days and, depending on individual risk level and need, a new Plan of Care will be developed and implemented.

9. Clients receiving the Postpartum Infant Universal Home Risk Assessment and meeting the following high-risk infant admission criteria are admitted to the Maternal/Newborn Home Care Program.
   a. The infant's birth weight is 1500 grams or less.
   b. The mother is 17 years old or younger.
   c. There has been inadequate prenatal care.
   d. The mother or infant has tested positive in a urine drug screen (UDS) or has tested positive for alcohol or drug abuse.
   e. Mother or infant suffers from immunosuppression.
   f. Medical necessity dictates home care. The reason must be specified (i.e., Apgar at 5 minutes <5, respiratory distress syndrome [RDS; mechanical vent >6 hours], intracranial hemorrhage, major congenital anomalies, central nervous system (CNS) infection or trauma, hyperbilirubinemia [>25 mg/dl], neonatal seizures, gastroesophageal reflux, congenitally acquired infection or disease, intensive care nursery, or another medical or social necessity determined by the pediatric health care provider).

10. Any problems identified will be reported to the health care provider. A Plan of Care will be developed for clients with the admission criteria listed above. Clients not meeting the admission criteria will have a community service plan developed by the health care provider or OB care coordinator.

11. As part of the screening, the nurse will complete both the physical and psychosocial risk assessments to help identify client needs for services in the home and community. Postpartum/Infant Risk Assessment Standards should be used to assure objectivity and to maximize use of services.

12. Levels of care
    After the initial evaluation, a Plan of Care will be developed in compliance with Medicare standards. The goals and objectives of the plan are based on the individual client's needs as identified by the screening.

    As part of the risk assessment section of the tool, the problems are assigned corresponding identifiers indicating a suggested level of care (i.e., a, cultural beliefs; b, inadequate food; c, current/recent abuse of drugs). These levels provide guidelines by which the agency, health care provider, client, and insurer can realistically plan for home care service need, directing the greatest intensity toward the greatest risks for poor outcome or preventable hospitalization. One rating (or more) in the next level requires that the client receive the higher level of care. For example, a client scoring all 1's would be at minimal risk, requiring level 1 services. If the client scored all 1's and a 2, that client would be at moderate risk and would therefore require level 2 services.

    Initial plan guidelines include the following:

    a. Level 1: One to three visits per month for the first 62 days. If meeting high-risk admission criteria, the client will be reevaluated every 62 days through the infant's first year, unless discharged.
    b. Level 2: One to three visits per week for the first 62 days. If meeting high-risk admission criteria, the client will be reevaluated every 62 days through the infant's first year, unless discharged.
    c. Level 3: Four to seven visits per week for the first 62 days. If meeting high-risk admission criteria, the client will be reevaluated every 62 days through the infant's first year, unless discharged.

13. Clients are discharged if the goals set are met or for one of the following reasons:
    a. There are no identified admission criteria justifying home care.
    b. The admission criterion problem has been identified and resolved at the initial visit.
    c. The goals in the established Plan of Care have been met.
    d. The goals cannot be met and the reasons are justified.

POSTPARTUM/INFANT PSYCHOSOCIAL STANDARDS FOR RISK ASSESSMENT

1. Life transitions: Life events that result in the possibility of changes in lifestyle, perceptions, behaviors, or belief systems.
   a. Denial or rejection of pregnancy: *Denial* is defined on a cognitive and emotional level as not acknowledging/accepting the pregnancy. *Rejection* is defined as a strong negative emotional or behavioral response to being pregnant.
   b. Past/current/recent incest or rape victim: Any evidence of sexual abuse or assault (incest or rape).
   c. History of infant/child chronic disability: Any diagnosed chronic physical or mental disability of another child.
   d. History of fetal death or other infant or pregnancy loss: Any loss that has occurred prenatally or within the infant's first year of life.
   e. Adoption or termination considered: Family seriously considering adoption or termination.

f. Suspected domestic violence: Suspected battering of child, parent or guardian, or both. Possible law enforcement involvement.

2. Emotional status: Identifiable affect (demeanor, emotional tones), mental status (intellectual functions; use of defenses; orientation to place, person, time), or emotional status (emotional control, emotional appropriateness) of patient or significant other.

   a. History of mental illness, mental health treatment, or hospitalization: Diagnosis of mental illness that may have included outpatient treatment.

   b. Unresolved grief or significant loss: Inability to reach acceptance in dealing with significant losses such as death of significant other; loss of job, home, or financial security; divorce or loss of relationship with significant other.

   c. Suicidal ideation: Serious suicidal tendencies as indicated by verbal threats, extreme depressed states, history of previous suicide attempts, and an actual suicide plan.

   d. Feelings of isolation, loneliness, or having inadequate support system: Expression of extreme loneliness. Patient may have family members or significant other present, but these people may provide insufficient or no emotional or financial support. Patient may not have any support.

   e. Questionable coping: Difficulties in adjusting to and accepting social relationships, life opportunities, activities of daily living (ADLs), and self-concept.

   f. History of depression: Evidence of a debilitating postpartum depression after a previous pregnancy (e.g., inability to take care of personal needs or even a single task, inability to bond or care for the child, potential abuse or neglect of self or infant).

   g. Evidence of low self-esteem: Verbal or nonverbal expression of low self-esteem, evidenced by lack of eye contact, downgrading one's self, disheveled appearance, withdrawal, negative self-concept.

3. Substance abuse or risk-taking behavior: Ongoing use or abuse of substances and evidence of risky behavior (e.g., multiple sex partners, no birth control method, tobacco use, behavioral problems in general).

   a. Current or recent abuse of alcohol: Ongoing use or use within past year of alcohol as it impacts on the individual and family. Includes those with no recent abuse but still living with other abusers.

   b. Current or recent abuse of street drugs: Ongoing use or use within past year of illicit drugs (e.g., heroin, marijuana, cocaine, barbiturates, amphetamines) or a referral from a drug abuse program. History of use or continuing abuse as it impacts on the individual and family. Includes those with no recent abuse but still living with other abusers.

   c. Current or recent use or abuse of prescribed medication: Ongoing use or use within past year of prescribed medication as it impacts on the individual and family. Includes those with no recent abuse but still living with other abusers.

   d. Law enforcement involvement: Law enforcement involvement with regard to impact on the parent's ability to access care or to care for the child.

   e. Sexual risk-taking behaviors: Includes but is not limited to multiple sex partners, no method of birth control, and unsafe sex practices. Includes those who live in crack houses.

   f. Tobacco use or secondhand smoke exposure: Ongoing use of tobacco (cigarettes, chewing tobacco, snuff) by the patient and its impact on the risk of secondhand smoke exposure to the infant or other children.

4. Parenting issues (observed or expressed): A client's perception of himself or herself in the role of parent in relation to the actual behaviors that are observed or expressed by the client.
   a. Teenaged or inexperienced parents: The particular developmental stage of the parent and how it impacts the ability to parent or nurture the child. Examples: a child raising a child, or an inexperienced parent exhibiting lack of confidence and fears regarding the ability to meet the needs of the child.
   b. Developmental issues (child or family expectations): Lack of knowledge or poor understanding of what is age-appropriate for the developing child. Inappropriate expectations may lead to punitive responses. Example: expecting an 18-month-old to toilet train and then punishing the child if there are continued "accidents."
   c. Discipline issues: Discipline methods are often culturally learned behaviors. Problems can occur when discipline is not appropriate to the child's developmental stage. Example: disciplining a crying 3-month-old because the child is perceived as being bad and deliberately crying to upset the parents.
   d. Relationship issues (bonding or nurturing): Poor eye contact, coldness, mother unable to cuddle with child (which can lead to failure to thrive).
   e. History of child abuse or neglect, now resolved: History of placement of other children due to abuse or neglect, currently resolved.
   f. Child abuse or neglect, or current child protective service involvement: Uncertainty regarding the possibility of abuse or neglect and anyone with current child protective service involvement. The staff person who directly observes possible abuse or neglect is required by law to report this. Assure interdisciplinary involvement and follow-up.
   g. Three or more children younger than 6 years of age: The possibility of increased stress related to the care of multiple young children with little support or few social outlets.

5. Educational or cultural barriers: These are potential barriers that are associated with greater than average infant mortality and morbidity or that might impede the patient's ability to follow instructions, meet expectations, or adhere to a recommended Plan of Care. Referrals might enhance the likelihood of appropriate use of services.
   a. Low literacy or limited intellectual ability: Evidence of inability or difficulty in reading basic instructions. Documentation of low or borderline intellectual capabilities.
   b. Language barriers: Inability to communicate basic information in English; also includes hearing and speech impairments.
   c. Cognitive deficits: Documented or perceived deficits in the ability to process information.
   d. Parent or guardian has not completed school beyond grade 12.
   e. Parent or guardian has not completed school beyond grade 10.
   f. Parent or guardian has not completed school beyond grade 9.
   g. Culture or beliefs: Cultural factors and beliefs that may impact health attitudes and behaviors, such as religious beliefs and practices, health values, attitudes toward getting and receiving health care, and present behaviors and lifestyle. These factors will vary among communities and individuals, and providers should be prepared to identify and respond to the needs of the populations they serve. Examples: cereal in an infant's bottle, jewelry for the baby, socks to cure hiccups, and coffee grounds to treat conjunctivitis.

6. Economic or resource needs: These factors could be appropriately handled through case management or, if more than one factor presents significant stress, through psychosocial intervention.
   a. Insufficient income or no income to meet basic needs.
   b. No transportation: Inability to secure adequate transportation to meet instrumental ADLs. This may include a child or family member's inability to plan or to take responsibility for required decision-making.
   c. Inadequate food: Difficulty in obtaining food to meet basic nutritional needs. May include lack of resources to purchase food or lack of knowledge about available resources.
   d. Legal needs: Need for assistance from the legal system (e.g., child support, divorce, domestic violence). May include lack of resources to secure legal aid or empowerment to effectively access available legal resources.
   e. Chronic difficulty accessing system: Persistent inability to access multiple agencies to assist with resources, impairing the ability to meet the most basic needs.
   f. Child care problems: Problems securing adequate acceptable child care such that gaining employment or accessing medical care is difficult or of low priority.
   g. Medicaid or general medical insurance problems: No existing permanent medical coverage for medical condition.

7. Maternal medical/nutritional factors
   a. Abnormal physical findings during this assessment: Any abnormal findings as noted on page 1 of the assessment tool.
   b. Problems with the chosen family planning method: The patient is unable to use the existing family planning methods successfully. Reasons may be medical, social, financial, religious, or emotional.
   c. Short interconceptual period: A period of less than 1 year between this conception and the preceding delivery.
   d. Grand multigravida: The patient has been pregnant more than seven times.
   e. Anemia: Hemoglobin < 10.8. If the patient does not know, ask if folic acid has been prescribed.
   f. Chronic disease: Medically diagnosed and documented chronic disease (e.g., diabetes, hypertension, renal disease, cardiovascular disease, liver disease, tuberculosis, sickle cell disease or trait, cancer, seizure disorder).
   g. HIV/AIDS: Any patient or significant other who has tested positive for the AIDS virus or has been medically diagnosed with the disease.
   h. Problem initiating breastfeeding: Any failed attempt at breastfeeding.
   i. Pica: Eating substances not ordinarily considered to be edible or to have nutritive value (e.g., dirt, clay, laundry starch).
   j. Anorexia/bulimia/fad diets: Suspected or medically diagnosed and documented case of anorexia/bulimia or other eating disorders; fad diets (e.g., grapefruit diet, diet pills).

8. Infant medical or nutritional factors
   a. Abnormal physical findings on this assessment: Any abnormal findings as noted in item 1 of the Infant Assessment Tool.

b. Prenatal exposure to drugs or alcohol: Maternal use of drugs and/or alcohol during pregnancy.

c. Infant anemia: hemoglobin <14.5 for a newborn, <9 for a 2-month-old, <11.5 for a 6- to 12-year-old.

d. Failure to thrive in siblings, previous or existing: Suspected or medically diagnosed and documented history and/or current condition.

e. Diagnosed or suspected malabsorption: Suspected or medically diagnosed and documented disorders (e.g., inadequate absorption of nutrients caused by one or combination of the following: infections, routine enteropathy, pancreatic insufficiency, gastric resection, antibiotic therapy, etc.).

f. Symptoms of intolerance to formula: An infant with overt symptoms of formula intolerance may present with any or all of these problems:

   1) Diarrhea (watery, large, frequent bowel movements that have a bad odor)

   2) Vomiting (throwing up large amounts of the stomach contents through the mouth)

   3) Constipation (painful bowel movements that are difficult to pass and look like small, hard balls)

   4) Abdominal distention

   5) Rash

   6) Bloody stools

   7) Other babies may present with milder symptoms similar to those of overt formula intolerance:

      (a) Spitting up

      (b) Gas

      (c) Fussiness

g. Gastroesophageal (GE) reflux: Medically diagnosed and documented GE reflux.

h. Low birth weight infant: Weight less than 2500 grams at birth.

i. Very low birth weight infant: Weight less than 1500 grams at birth.

j. Inadequate prenatal care: Less than four prenatal visits, for any reason.

k. Previous hospitalization of siblings in first year.

l. Extended neonatal intensive care unit (NICU) hospitalization: Neonatal course for the child that includes treatment and more than an overnight stay for observation in the NICU.

m. Medical problems related to prematurity: Any medical problem, current or residual, as a result of birth at or before 37 weeks.

n. Medical problems related to congenital anomalies: Any medical problem, current or residual, as a result of any congenital anomaly.

o. Sexually transmitted disease (STD) exposure in pregnancy, untreated: Documented STD, untreated or treatment not completed. Includes chlamydia, herpes, syphilis, gonorrhea, HIV, and hepatitis.

p. Lead exposure: An answer of "yes" to any of the following risk-assessment questions means the child is at risk:

1) Does your child live in or regularly visit a house built before 1960? Is/was your child's day care center/preschool/home built before 1960? Do any of these dwellings have peeling or chipping paint?
2) Does your child live in a house built before 1960 with recent, ongoing, or planned renovation or remodeling?
3) Have any of your children or their playmates had lead poisoning?
4) Does your child frequently come in contact with an adult who works with lead? Examples are construction, welding, pottery, or other trades practiced in your community.
5) Does you child live near a lead smelter, battery recycling plant, or other industry likely to release lead into the community? Cite other examples.
6) Do you give your child any home or folk remedies that may contain lead?
7) Does your child live near a heavily traveled major highway where soil or dust may be contaminated with lead?
8) Does your home's plumbing have lead pipes or copper with lead solder joints?

8. Environmental problems
   a. Housing problems: Includes any of the following:
      1) Living space or accommodations inadequate for the number of occupants in the household, indicating that a potential health or safety hazard exists.
      2) Conditions that are substandard, indicating that clear safety hazards exist (e.g., poor sanitation, ventilation, heating, electrical hazards, vector infestation).
      3) Movement from one house/apartment/shelter to another without a stable home base or a network of support systems. This could include the migrant population.
      4) Without housing, totally reliant on community support for shelter, or living on the streets.
   b. Utilities: Lack of electricity, heat, phone, or air conditioning in those situations where they are basic necessities.
   c. Water/sewer: Lack of water/sewer.
   d. Refrigeration: Lack of refrigeration.
   e. Unsafe neighborhood: Neighborhood is an area of high crime or otherwise known to be unsafe for its residents. This would include a known drug area.
   f. Inadequate preparation for infant: Lack of preparation for meeting the basic needs of a newborn in the home (e.g., no crib, car seat, clothing, formula).

PHYSICAL STANDARDS: STANDARDS OF CARE—MATERNAL ASSESSMENT

1. Temperature
   a. *Standards within normal limits (WNL):* Oral temperature should be between 97°F and 100.3°F.
   b. *Deviations:* Oral temperature above 100.4°F is notable.

c. *Evaluation of deviations:* It is not unusual for the mother's temperature to rise to 100.4°F in the first 24 hours after delivery if unaccompanied by other symptoms. If her temperature elevates after 24 hours and persists for 48 hours, it is abnormal. Check for other symptoms such as foul-smelling lochia, calf or leg pain, undue pain or discomfort, or burning upon urination.

d. *Action:* If her temperature is between 99°F and 100.4°F, check for breast engorgement. If her temperature is 100.4°F, assess for mastitis, endometritis, urinary tract infection, or other systemic infection. Call the health care provider from the client's home and relate your findings if infection is suspected. If infection is *not* suspected, instruct the mother in the signs and symptoms of infection, then retake her temperature every 4 hours. She should report to her health care provider any of the following: signs and symptoms of infection, persistent temperature elevation over 24 hours, or a temperature higher than 100.4°F.

2. Pulse

   a. *Standards WNL:* Pulse rate should be between 50 and 90 bpm.

   b. *Deviations:* A pulse rate less than 50 or greater than 100 bpm is abnormal.

   c. *Evaluation of deviations:* Pulse rate falls a short time after delivery and bradycardia may persist for 6 to 8 days. Pulse rates greater than 90 bpm could indicate either infection or hypovolemic shock if other signs have also deviated from the norm (e.g., hypotension, increased amounts of vaginal bleeding, diaphoresis, or pallor).

   d. *Action:* If the pulse rate is greater than 90 bpm and other signs are evident, call health care provider from the client's home immediately and relate your findings.

3. Blood pressure

   a. *Standards WNL:* Blood pressure should remain in accord with previous readings if there were no problems. A good range is 90/60 to 140/90. Deviations must be measured against the average blood pressure of the individual client. A history of blood pressure must be obtained from client.

   b. *Deviations:* The following are abnormal findings: a sustained rise of 30 mm Hg or more in systolic blood pressure, a sustained rise of 15 mm Hg or more in diastolic blood pressure, a sustained systolic blood pressure of 140 mm Hg or more, or a sustained diasystolic blood pressure of 90 mm Hg or more.

   c. *Evaluation of deviations:* There is a small risk of postpartum toxemia until the cardiovascular system is relieved of the excess fluid volume normally acquired in pregnancy. Evaluate to determine if edema and headache are present. Hypotension can be a late sign of hypovolemic shock; other signs are usually evident before a decrease in blood pressure. Orthostatic hypotension can occur in the first 48 hours but should not persist unless some underlying condition is present.

   d. *Action:* If the patient has an increase in blood pressure along with blurred vision, headache, and edema, call her health care provider immediately. If other symptoms are not present, take blood pressure in both arms. If the elevated pressure is evident in both arms, have the client lie down for 15 minutes and retake her blood pressure. If the patient has decreased blood pressure and is asymptomatic, instruct the client to notify her health care provider if she becomes symptomatic.

4. Perineum

   a. *Standards WNL:* The episiotomy should be dry and intact; some discomfort is normal.

   b. *Deviations:* Swollen, bruised perineum accompanied by extreme pain and possible foul-smelling discharge is notable.

c. *Evaluation of deviations:* Increased perineal pain can be indicative of a vaginal hematoma. Obtain labor and delivery history and assess perineal area closely for swollen or bruised areas. Check for intact episiotomy and for other signs/symptoms of infection, such as elevated temperature and foul-smelling discharge.

d. *Action:* Notify the health care provider from the client's home if the client is having extreme pain that is not relieved by normal techniques such as sitz bath and analgesics. Notify the health care provider also if the episiotomy appears swollen and if discharge is foul smelling. Encourage the client to cleanse perineal area from front to back and to use good handwashing technique.

5. Gastrointestinal system

a. *Standards WNL:* The client should have well-formed brown stool by second or third postpartum day or fourth day following cesarean section.

b. *Deviations:* Nonexistent bowel sounds or the inability to have a bowel movement by third day following delivery should be investigated.

c. *Evaluation of deviations:* During labor or any operative procedure such as cesarean section birth, peristalsis ceases. Auscultate for bowel sounds in client. Obtain a history of the client's normal bowel pattern.

d. *Action:* If bowel sounds are nonexistent, encourage increased ambulation and a liquid diet until the client feels gas movement. If this does not occur within 24 hours, instruct the client to notify the health care provider. If bowel sounds are present but the client has not moved bowels, exercise, increased roughage in diet, and increased fluids are recommended. Instruct the client to notify her health care provider if there has been no bowel movement by the fifth day following delivery, or sooner if uncomfortable.

6. Fundus or uterus

a. *Standards WNL:* The fundus should be firm and should be positioned 1 to 2 centimeters above the umbilicus, down to 3 centimeters below the umbilicus.

b. *Deviations:* The following are abnormal findings: soft fundal tone, failure to contract after massage, evident increased vaginal bleeding, or fundus positioned 3 to 4 centimeters above umbilicus with right deviation.

c. *Evaluation of deviations:* Determine the intrapartum course for evidence of retained placenta, large neonate, multiple gestation, or grand multipara. Massage fundus gently. Overstimulation of the fundus can cause inversion of uterus. Instruct the client to massage fundus. Check the amount of vaginal bleeding. Check for urinary retention. Consult with the health care provider. Uterus displaced to the right usually indicates bladder distension due to inadequate urination. Evaluate urinary status.

d. *Action:* Notify the health care provider immediately from the client's home if the fundus remains soft and increased vaginal bleeding persists. Use techniques to induce urination (running water, sitz bath, etc.). Make certain that the client is aware that she should contact her health care provider if she has any difficulties in voiding.

7. Lochia

a. *Standards WNL:* Presence of a moderate ($^1/_2$ to $^3/_4$ pad) amount of dark red blood for initial 2 to 3 days is normal. Odor should be that of normal menstrual flow (Jacobsen, 1985).

b. *Deviations:* If lochia is excessive, with fully saturated pads of bright red blood after 1 to 2 hours, or is foul smelling, it should be investigated.

c. *Evaluation of deviations:* Obtain a detailed labor and delivery history. Encourage the client to keep a record of pads used and saturation status. Determine whether other signs and symptoms are evident that would indicate abnormal involution (e.g., atonic uterus, hypotension, tachycardia). Foul-smelling lochia is indicative of infection. Check temperature for two consecutive readings of 100.4°F or higher. Check for tiredness.

d. *Action:* Check the client's fundus for tone. Check episiotomy for intactness. Check the consistency and amount of bleeding. If it is excessive, compare with other signs and symptoms and notify the health care provider immediately from client's home if necessary. If temperature is 100.4°F or higher for two consecutive readings or if there is a foul-smelling lochia, call the health care provider from the client's home.

8. Urinary system

   a. *Standards WNL:* Output should be 1500 ml per 24-hour period via urinary tract.

   b. *Deviations:* Decreased output of less than 30 ml per hour, dysuria, frequent urination with small amounts, or pain with chills and fever, all are abnormal findings.

   c. *Evaluation of deviations:* Evaluate the client's voiding patterns. Determine if the client had any difficulty voiding in the hospital and if her health care provider was aware of this. Evaluate the fundal height to verify bladder distention. Check the client's temperature.

   d. *Action:* Notify the health care provider from the client's home if signs and symptoms of urinary tract infection or bladder distention are present.

9. Breasts

   a. *Standards WNL:* Two mammary glands with wide, pigmented areolas are normal. Sometimes there is a less-pigmented area called the secondary areola. Venous engorgement may be visible along with striations of the skin. The nipple is erect and deeply pigmented. Some patients may have flat or inverted nipples. Breastfeeding should be encouraged and supported as a method of feeding. Breasts of nonnursing mothers will become full and the mother may experience moderate discomfort.

   b. *Deviations:* A duct of the breast may become clogged, causing the milk to back up. The area becomes tender to the touch and reddened, and infection can set in. An elevated temperature accompanies this condition. Another problem that may arise is breast engorgement. Also, the nursing mother's breasts may not fill adequately. Try to ensure that an adequate breastfeeding pattern is established. Sore nipples may also cause discomfort for the nursing mother.

   c. *Evaluation of deviations:* If a breast duct becomes clogged, evaluate for signs and symptoms of mastitis: chills, fever, malaise, axillary adenopathy, extremely tender breast, cracked nipples, plugged milk ducts. For engorged breasts, determine the method of feeding. If breastfeeding, evaluate the hardness of the breast and the ability of the infant to latch onto the nipple. Check for discomfort, as well as for signs and symptoms of mastitis. If you suspect that the mother's breasts are not filling adequately, check if the breasts are soft to the touch after the third postpartum day before scheduled infant feed. Evaluate the mother's hydration, pattern of feeding, and whether supplements are offered. If her breasts are inadequately filling, the mother may complain of a constantly hungry infant. For sore nipples, reassure the client that nipples often become sore initially. Evaluate the interference with breastfeeding establishment.

d. *Action:* Notify the health care provider from the client's home when mastitis is present so that antibiotics may be ordered. Encourage the client to maintain breastfeeding on the affected side. Place warm compresses on the reddened area. Do not stop breastfeeding or pumping. This could aggravate the condition. In a nonnursing mother, instruct the client to wear supportive bra and to apply ice to breast. Avoid any stimulation to breasts (shower backwards). Acetaminophen may be taken on advice from the health care provider. Instruct the client in the signs and symptoms of infection. She should report these to her health care provider. If her breasts are not filling adequately, establish the following plan with the mother to promote breastfeeding. No supplements should be offered before 2 hours of anticipated feed. Always offer the breast first to satiate infant's hunger. Allow the infant to suckle 15 minutes each side. Positions should be changed each feed to minimize nipple soreness. Breastfeed every 2 to 3 hours; avoid overexhaustion. For the exhausted mother: Breastfeed only 5 minutes each side and go back to sleep immediately. A support person may feed the infant formula supplement if indicated. The support person should feed and care for the infant away from the mother's sleeping area. If the mother has sore nipples, instruct her to persist, because the soreness will resolve. Change the infant's positions with each feeding (lying down, football, sitting up, cradle, semireclining with infant facing mother). Always allow the nipples to dry thoroughly (may blow dry from safe distance). Use warm, sterile saltwater soaks; apply Eucerin cream (Masse contains alcohol, which may irritate) to areola (do not plug nipple opening with any cream) or radiant heat from household light bulb directed toward nipple (not over 60 watts). Offer a breastfeeding counselor to all breastfeeding mothers.

10. Psychological status

    a. *Standards WNL:* The beginning maternal–infant bond has formed. Emotional fluctuations may be evident but should resolve by the fourth postpartum day.

    b. *Deviations:* Postpartum psychosis, detachment from infant, and maladjustment to body image changes are all reasons for concern.

    c. *Evaluation of deviations:* Evaluate for signs of postpartum psychosis such as infant detachment, disinterest in personal appearance and nutrition, anxiety, anorexia, and exaggerated fatigue. The mother may express strange or inappropriate thoughts or feelings, delusions, hallucinations, or hostility toward significant other and medical staff.

    d. *Action:* Consult with the health care provider for the best plan of action. Emphasize the need for follow-up visitation, especially for safe caretaking of the newborn.

STANDARDS OF CARE FOR INFANT ASSESSMENT

1. Skin

    a. *Standards within normal limits (WNL):* Skin color should be pink and the skin should be warm to touch; some mottling may be present in extremities. A slightly yellow color with blanching about nose or the presence of a normal newborn rash, birthmark, or mongolian spots is also a normal finding.

    b. *Deviations:* Evidence of cyanosis about face or lips requires investigation; the infant who appears very pale or ruddy should be evaluated. Icterus, a yellow skin tone to blanching about face and abdomen, is also an abnormal finding. Another finding to investigate is a rash appearing to be spreading out from inside the anus. Any rash characterized by bright red papules that may erupt and form craterlike ulcers or that appears to contain pustules is cause for further assessment.

c. *Evaluation of deviations:* Observe the degree of cyanosis while the infant is eating or crying. Evaluate the activity level, vital signs, heart and lung sounds, effect of posturing infant, suck, interest and ability to maintain time needed to feed. If there is evidence of icterus, determine if bilirubin was drawn in the hospital and if the mother had instructions for follow-up. Determine, if possible, the mother's and infant's blood types. (If the mother is type O, determine if she received RhoGAM; report immediately to the health care provider if the baby has a positive blood type and the mother did not receive RhoGAM). Evaluate the infant's activity level, interest in feeds, color of stools, and the presence of yellow in sclera. If the baby has a suspicious rash, evaluate the maternal history of infection and the length of time from rupture of membrane (ROM). Assess other vital signs and check for signs and symptoms of infection in the infant. Determine if the baby's health care provider is aware of the rash and what treatment has been prescribed.

d. *Action:* If infant's skin tone is yellow to blanching about abdomen or if sclera appears yellow, assess the infant and notify the health care provider from the client's home. If the infant is slightly yellow only about the face, is active, alert, and eating well, instruct the mother to provide extra water after feeds and with signs and symptoms of jaundice (yellow about abdomen or sclera, lethargy, decreased interest in feeds). The family should be aware to notify the health care provider if the signs and symptoms increase. If the infant has a rash and is not under the health care provider's care, notify the health care provider of your findings from the client's home.

2. Head

a. *Standards WNL:* A rounded head is normal; some molding may be apparent. Axillary temperature should be between 97°F and 99°F.

b. *Deviations:* Caput succedaneum, which may cross cranial sutures, merits further evaluation. Cephalhematoma, which does not cross cranial sutures, is also an abnormal finding. If the infant is unable to move his or her head from side to side, it may indicate neurologic trauma. Asymmetrical flattened occiput on either side of head may indicate plagiocephaly. If the infant holds his or her head at an angle, torticollis is a possibility. An axillary temperature below 97°F or above 99°F, or swings of more than 2°F from one reading to the next are also abnormal findings.

c. *Evaluation of deviations:* If you suspect caput succedaneum or cephalhematoma, evaluate the infant's neurologic reflexes. Evaluate for signs and symptoms of intracranial hemorrhage (abnormal respiration with cyanosis, shrill cry, reduced responsiveness, tense fontanelle, and convulsions—twitching of the lower jaw with salivation is often a sign of convulsion). If head movement, asymmetrical flattened occiput, or the head's angle is a problem, instruct the parents to change the infant's sleeping positions frequently and call the health care provider if there is no improvement.

For temperature problems, keep in mind that infant temperature may rise to 100.2°F or decrease to 96.6°F if the infant is exposed to excessive warmth or chill. The infant should be wrapped or unwrapped according to temperature deviation. Retake the child's temperature in 15 minutes. Evaluate the infant for signs and symptoms of sepsis or other infection (poor suck, anorexia, regurgitation of feeds, diarrhea, jaundice, pallor, cyanosis, tremors, lethargy, hyper- or hyporeflexes, bradypnea, petechiae). Review the maternal history of infections and length of time from rupture of membrane. Teach the parents to use a thermometer. Assess their ability to read the thermometer.

d. *Action:* Educate the parents that caput and cephalhematoma will resolve. Contact the health care provider if signs or symptoms of intracranial hemorrhage or neurologic problems are suspected. If head movement, asymmetrical flattened occiput, or the head's angle is a problem, document the condition for the health care provider to review at the first well-baby visit. For the infant with a temperature, if a rise and fall of temperature does not occur and the infant is free of signs and symptoms of infection and other vital signs are WNL, the mother should retake the child's temperature in 1 hour and call the health care provider if there is no improvement. If signs and symptoms of sepsis or any type of infection are present, the nurse must call the health care provider from the client's home. If the child's temperature is below 96.6°F or above 100.2°F, call the health care provider immediately. Call the health care provider if the child's temperature swings 2°F or more from one reading to next.

3. Neck

   a. *Standards WNL:* Short, straight creases with skin folds are normal. The posterior neck lacks loose extra folds of skin. The head should move freely from side to side.

   b. *Deviations:* An abnormally short neck is cause for further investigation. The following conditions also require attention: arching or inability to flex the neck (meningitis, congenital anomaly, webbing of neck, Turner's syndrome, Down's syndrome, trisomy 18) and neck rigidity (congenital torticollis, 11th nerve damage).

   c. *Evaluation of deviations:* Collect more data indicative of chromosomal aberrations. Determine the maternal history of infections and length of time from rupture of membrane. Assess the infant for signs of infection.

   d. *Action:* If a congenital defect is suspected, contact the health care provider and the agency for consultation outside of the client's home. If the infant evidences signs or symptoms of infection, contact the health care provider from the client's home.

4. Eyes

   a. *Standards WNL:* The cornea and retina should be clear. The ability to follow a light with the eyes is notable.

   b. *Deviations:* Ulceration (herpes infection), large cornea or corneas of unequal size (congenital glaucoma), or clouding, opacity of lens (cataract) are all abnormal findings.

   c. *Evaluation of deviations:* Determine the history of maternal infection and the length of time from rupture of membrane. Determine whether the health care provider is aware of the deviation.

   d. *Action:* Contact the health care provider from the client's home unless the mother indicates that the baby is already under treatment by the health care provider for the deviation.

5. Pupils

   a. *Standards WNL:* The pupils should be equal in size and round, and should react to light by accommodation.

   b. *Deviations:* Abnormal findings include unequal pupils (central nervous system damage), dilatation or constriction (intracranial damage, retinoblastoma, glaucoma), and pupils that are nonreactive to light or accommodation (brain injury).

   c. *Evaluation of deviations:* Assess neurologic reflexes.

   d. *Action:* Report your findings to the baby's health care provider from the client's home.

6. Conjunctiva

   a. *Standards WNL:* Chemical conjunctivitis (subsides in 2 to 7 days), palpebral conjunctiva (red, not hyperemic), and subconjunctival hemorrhage are all within normal limits.

   b. *Deviations:* The following conditions are not within normal limits: pale color (anemia), inflammation or edema, purulent drainage (infection, blocked tear duct).

   c. *Evaluation of deviations:* Determine the history of maternal infections and the length of time from rupture of membrane. Determine the history of eye drainage and whether under treatment by a health care provider for the deviation.

   d. *Action:* Contact the health care provider from the client's home if the baby is not under treatment for the deviation.

7. Eyes/vision

   a. *Standards WNL:* The infant should be able to track moving object to midline. The ability to follow a light with the eyes is notable.

   b. *Deviations:* Cataracts (congenital) or infections are abnormal findings.

   c. *Evaluation of deviations:* Determine the history of maternal infections during pregnancy.

   d. *Action:* Record any questions about visual activity for the health care provider to follow up at the first well-baby check-up.

8. General appearance

   a. *Standards WNL:* Eyes should be bright and clear, evenly placed, with slight nystagmus, concomitant strabismus, and should move in all directions. At birth, eyes are blue-slate in color, or brown in babies of color.

   b. *Deviations:* Gross nystagmus (damage to the third, fourth, and sixth cranial nerves), constant and fixed strabismus, lack of pigmentation (albinism), and Brushfield's spots (may indicate Down's syndrome) are all abnormal findings. "Sunset eyes," ptosis, and an upward slant in nonorientals should be investigated as well.

   c. *Evaluation of deviations:* Determine what information was given to the mother in the hospital. Do not upset the family with only suspected defects. Call the health care provider and the agency for consultation from your home prior to presenting your suspicions to family. Evaluate neurologic status.

   d. *Action:* Indicate to the parent that you will call your report in to the health care provider. Call the health care provider and the agency from your home. Follow the instructions of the health care provider and the agency.

9. Ears

   a. *Standards WNL:* Ears should be well formed. They may have minor anomalies such as auricular fistulas and tubercles. A twisted or rotated ear may give the false impression of being low set.

   b. *Deviations:* Gross malformations or low-set ears are not within normal limits.

   c. *Evaluation of deviations:* Evaluate the setting of the ears by holding a pen or pencil from the outer canthus of the eye. This should give a straight appearance, as if wearing glasses.

   d. *Action:* Identify with the parent if the health care provider is aware of the deviation. Report to the physician from the client's home if the parent states that the health care provider is unaware of the deviation.

10. Nose/external nasal aspects
    a. *Standards WNL:* The nose may appear flattened as a result of delivery process. Patent nares bilaterally.
    b. *Deviations:* A continued flat or broad bulge of nose (Down's syndrome) or blockage of the nares (mucus or secretions) is abnormal.
    c. *Evaluation of deviations:* Assess for signs and symptoms of infection.
    d. *Action:* Consult with physician from your home if you suspect a congenital defect. If signs and symptoms of infection are present, contact the health care provider from the client's home. If there are no signs and symptoms of infection, instruct in the use of a bulb syringe if available. The family should contact the health care provider if the problem persists.
11. Nose/internal aspects
    a. *Standards WNL:* Pink and firm mucous membranes are within normal limits. The septum should be midline and without polyps or tumors.
    b. *Deviations:* A deviated or perforated septum, or tumors or polyps of the septum are abnormal findings. Swelling and erythema also are notable.
    c. *Evaluation of deviations:* Determine the infant's ability to make good air exchange, auscultate lungs, and assess restlessness and irritability. Assess for signs and symptoms of infection or distress.
    d. *Action:* Determine if the baby's health care provider is following a deviation. Contact the provider from the client's home if the infant appears to experience any distress.
12. Mouth/function of facial, hypoglossopharyngeal, and vagus nerves
    a. *Standards WNL:* Symmetry of movement and strength are normal findings. Assess for adequate salivation, presence of gag, swallowing, and sucking reflexes. The tongue should be midline.
    b. *Deviations:* If the mouth draws to one side, it may indicate transient seventh cranial nerve paralysis due to pressure in utero or trauma during delivery or congenital paralysis. A fishlike shape may indicate Treacher Collins syndrome. Suppressed or absent reflexes are also abnormal. Deviations from midline could imply cranial nerve damage.
    c. *Evaluation of deviations:* Evaluate other neurologic functions.
    d. *Action:* Notify the health care provider from the client's home if the parent states that the provider is unaware of the deviation.
13. Palate (soft and hard)
    a. *Standards WNL:* The hard palate should be dome shaped and the uvula should be midline with symmetric movement of the soft palate. The palate should be intact, and the infant should suck well when stimulated. Epithelial (Epstein's) pearls often appear on mucosa.
    b. *Deviations:* A high-steepled palate could be a sign of Treacher Collins syndrome. Clefts in either the hard or soft palate may point to a polygenic disorder.
    c. *Evaluation of deviations:* Evaluate infant hydration, ability to feed, respiratory status, and parental bonding.
    d. *Action:* The infant with a cleft palate will be under a health care provider's care. Report the progress of the baby to the health care provider from the client's home.

14. Pharynx
    a. *Standards WNL:* The pharynx should be unobstructed, with no drainage in the back of the throat and no exudate on the tonsils. The esophagus should be patent; some drooling is common in newborns.
    b. *Deviations:* If exudate is present, it may be a sign of infection. Excessive drooling or bubbling may point to esophageal atresia.
    c. *Evaluation of deviations:* If exudate is present, examine for other signs of infection. For possible esophageal atresia, evaluate possible esophageal defects by reviewing the infant's feeding history.
    d. *Action:* Report all abnormal findings to the health care provider from the client' s home.

15. Tongue
    a. *Standards WNL:* The tongue should be free-moving in all directions and midline. It should have a pink color, with a smooth to rough texture, noncoated. The tongue should also be proportional to the mouth. Sucking and rooting reflexes should be present. The infant should be able to discriminate pleasant from unpleasant tastes.
    b. *Deviations:* The following are not within normal limits: Lack of movement or asymmetric movement, tongue-tied; white cheesy coating (thrush); deep ridges; a large tongue with short frenulum (cretinism, Down's and other mental retardation syndromes); and absence of reaction of tongue to various stimuli (seventh cranial nerve damage).
    c. *Evaluation of deviations:* If there is a lack of movement, further assess neurologic functions. Test reflexes, elevation of tongue when depressed with tongue blade. Check for signs of weakness or deviation. If there is a white coating, differentiate between thrush and milk curds. Reassure the parents that the tongue pattern may change from day to day. For all other deviations, evaluate neurologic status and assess neurologic functions.
    d. *Action:* Notify the health care provider from the client's home if a deviation or infection is suspected. Consult with the health care provider from your home whenever a congenital defect is suspected.

16. Gums
    a. *Standards WNL:* The gums should be dark pink, firm, and smooth. There will be a dark (melanotic) line along the gums in black babies.
    b. *Deviations:* Inflamed gums (infection), pallor (anemia), and precocious teeth should all be examined more closely.
    c. *Evaluation of deviations:* Evaluate for other signs and symptoms of anemia or infection.
    d. *Action:* Notify the health care provider from the client's home if anemia or infection is suspected.

17. Lips
    a. *Standards WNL:* Labial tubercle (pink, sucking blisters) is normal. Mucosa of lips should be well demarcated from the surrounding skin. Saliva should be scant. Lips fused in midline.
    b. *Deviations:* Cleft lip (polygenic disorder) and a thin upper lip require closer inspection.
    c. *Evaluation of deviations:* Counsel parents on special feeding techniques that may be necessary if the child has a cleft lip. Assess for fetal alcohol syndrome if the child has a thin upper lip.

   d. *Action:* For a cleft lip, parents should be aware to contact the health care provider if feeding problems persist. If the child has fetal alcohol syndrome, refer the family to an early intervention program.

18. Chest/clavicles

   a. *Standards WNL:* The clavicles should be straight and intact, the moro reflex should be elicitable, and there should be bilateral movement of both shoulders.

   b. *Deviations:* The following conditions require further examination: a knot or lump on clavicle (fracture during difficult delivery), or a unilateral moro reflex response on unaffected side (fracture of clavicle, brachial palsy, Erb–Duchenne syndrome).

   c. *Evaluation of deviations:* For a knot or lump on the clavicle, obtain a detailed labor and delivery history. Assess respiratory status.

   d. *Action:* Notify the health care provider from the client's home if a deviation is suspected that is not already diagnosed and under treatment.

19. Appearance and size of chest

   a. *Standards WNL:* The circumference should be 32.5 cm or 1 to 2 cm less than the head. The chest should be wider than it is long; it should be of a normal shape without depressed or prominent sternum. The lower end of the sternum (xiphoid cartilage) may be protruding; this is less apparent after several weeks. The sternum should be about 8 cm long.

   b. *Deviations:* Funnel chest (congenital or associated with Marfan's syndrome), continued protrusion of xiphoid cartilage (Marfan's syndrome; "pigeon chest"), and barrel chest are findings beyond normal limits.

   c. *Evaluation of deviations:* If Marfan's syndrome is suspected, measure at the level of the nipples after exhalation. For barrel chest, determine the adequacy of other respiratory and circulatory signs. Assess for other signs and symptoms of various syndromes.

   d. *Action:* Notify the health care provider from the client's home if a deviation is suspected or apparent.

20. Expansion and retraction

   a. *Standards WNL:* Bilateral expansion or no intracostal, subcostal, or suprasternal retraction are normal findings.

   b. *Deviations:* Unequal chest expansion (pneumonia, pneumothorax respiratory distress) and retractions (respiratory distress) are abnormal findings.

   c. *Evaluation of deviations:* Collect more data regarding respiratory effort if chest expansion is unequal (regulatory, flaring of nares, difficulty on both inspiration and expiration). If there are retractions, examine the chest thoroughly using the techniques of inspection, palpation, and auscultation.

   d. *Action:* Notify the health care provider from the client's home if a deviation is suspected or apparent.

21. Chest percussion

   a. *Standards WNL:* Decreased percussion over liver, diaphragm, and heart, with these areas well demarcated, is within normal limits.

   b. *Deviations:* Dullness in lung fields (consolidation of lungs, atelectasis) or hyperresonance of the chest (pneumonia, pneumothorax, distended stomach) should be evaluated further.

c. *Evaluation of deviations:* Examine the chest thoroughly using the techniques of inspection, palpation, and auscultation.

d. *Action:* Notify the health care provider from the client's home if a deviation is suspected or apparent.

22. Auscultation

a. *Standards WNL:* Breath sounds are louder in infants and heard bilaterally. The chest and axilla clear on crying.

b *Deviations:* Decreased breath sounds may indicate decreased respiratory activity, atelectasis, pneumothorax. Increased breath sounds are heard with resolving pneumonia.

c. *Evaluation of deviations:* Perform a complete physical exam and collaborate with the health care provider regarding positive findings.

d. *Action:* Notify the health care provider from the client's home if a deviation is suspected or apparent.

23. Respiratory rate

a. *Standards WNL:* The respiratory rate should be between 30 to 60 breaths per minute.

b. *Deviations:* A rate below 30 and above 60 requires follow up.

c. *Evaluation of deviations:* Assess the infant's entire respiratory status and observe color and activity level to determine adequate oxygenation. The infant with a respiratory rate between 20 and 30 breaths per minute may be receiving adequate oxygenation; the rate should increase with stimulation. A rate from 60 to 80 without other signs of distress may be due to increased activity (crying, etc.). Assess and collaborate with the health care provider if questionable.

d. *Action:* Notify the health care provider from the client's home of a rate below 20/minute or above 80/minute, or if any signs or symptoms of distress are noted, regardless of rate.

24. Bronchial breath sounds (heard when trachea and bronchi closest to chest wall, above sternum and between scapulae) and determination of point of maximal impulse (PMI)

a. *Standards WNL:* Bronchial sounds bilaterally. The air entry is clear. Rates may indicate normal newborn atelectasis. Cough reflex absent at birth, appears in 2 or more days. It is difficult to assess exact PMI in an infant under 2 years old, but usually at lateral to midclavicular line at third or fourth interspace.

b. *Deviations:* Adventitious or abnormal sounds (respiratory diseases or distress) and malpositioning (enlargement, abnormal placement, pneumothorax, dextrocardia, diaphragmatic hernia) require investigation.

c. *Evaluation of deviations:* Initiate cardiac and respiratory evaluation.

d. *Action:* Notify the health care provider from the client's home of any suspected deviation.

25. Breasts

a. *Standards WNL:* Breasts should be flat with symmetrical nipple. Breast tissue has a diameter of 5 cm or more at term. The distance between nipples is 8 cm. Breast engorgement occurs on the third day of life, and liquid discharge may be expressed in term infants.

b. *Deviations:* A lack of breast tissue may indicate prematurity or SGA (small for gestational age). Breast abscesses are not within the normal limits.

c. *Evaluation of deviations:* Reassure parents that breast engorgement is normal. Assess for signs and symptoms of infection.

d. *Action:* Notify the health care provider from the client's home of any deviations present or if a follow-up appointment is required sooner than the normal well-baby follow up, due to SGA, prematurity, or low birth weight.

26. Heart auscultation and palpation

    a. *Standards WNL:* The heart lies horizontally, with the left border extending to the left of midclavicle. There should be a regular rhythm and rate. Functional murmurs may be present, no thrills, with a split second sound (lub, splat). Heart rate should be 100 to 160.

    b. *Deviations:* Arrhythmia (anoxia), tachycardia, bradycardia are abnormal findings. Location of murmurs (possible congenital cardiac anomaly) also requires further study. Rates of 90 to 100 and 160 to 180 require evaluation for adequate oxygenation, good circulatory effort, increase or decrease with corresponding activity level. Respiratory rate should be within normal limits. Rates at 90 (sleeping) or at 180 (crying).

    c. *Evaluation of deviations:* Evaluate any murmur: location, timing, and duration; observe for accompanying cardiac pathology symptoms, and ascertain any family history.

    d. *Action:* All arrhythmia and gallop rhythms should be referred to the health care provider from the client's home. Report any evidence of circulatory compromise. Report to the health care provider any rate below 90 or above 180, even if the infant appears to be in no distress.

27. Trachea (palpate from top to bottom with thumb and index fingers)

    a. *Standards WNL:* The trachea should be slightly right of midline.

    b. *Deviations:* Deviated left or right (pneumothorax, tumor of chest or neck) is not within normal limits.

    c. *Evaluation of deviations:* Initiate cardiopulmonary evaluation.

    d. *Action:* Notify the health care provider from the client's home if a deviation is suspected.

28. Rib cage and diaphragm

    a. *Standards WNL:* A horizontal groove at the diaphragm shows flaring of the rib cage to a mild degree.

    b. *Deviations:* Harrison's groove with marked flaring indicates a vitamin D deficiency. Inadequacy of respiration movement requires further inquiry.

    c. *Evaluation of deviations:* Initiate cardiopulmonary evaluation.

    d. *Action:* Notify the health care provider from the client's home if a deviation is suspected.

29. Abdomen/appearance

    a. *Standards WNL:* The abdomen should be cylindrical with some protrusion and appear large in relation to pelvis; some laxness of abdominal muscles is normal. There should be no cyanosis and few vessels can be seen. Diastasis recti is common in black infants. Observe for synchronous movement with breathing.

    b. *Deviations:* A distended, shiny abdomen with engorged vessels may indicate gastrointestinal abnormalities, infection, or congenital megacolon. A scaphoid appearance may be evidence of a diaphragmatic hernia. Increased or decreased peristalsis needs to be evaluated. Localized flank bulging (enlarged kidneys, ascites, or absent abdominal muscles) also requires evaluation.

c. *Evaluation of deviations:* Examine abdomen thoroughly for mass or organomegaly. For localized flank bulging, assess for other signs and symptoms of obstruction.

d. Notify the health care provider from the client's home if a deviation is suspected or apparent.

30. Palpation

a. *Standards WNL:* The abdomen should be nontender with no palpable masses.

b. *Deviations:* A tense abdomen with marked rigidity or resistance to pressure may indicate infection. Solid mass (Wilms' tumor) or teratoma mass located below the umbilicus is abnormal finding.

c. *Evaluation of deviations:* Take temperature and assess other signs and symptoms.

d. *Action:* Notify the health care provider from the client's home if a deviation is suspected or apparent.

31. Umbilicus

a. *Standards WNL:* There should be no protrusion of umbilicus and no umbilical hernia; protrusion of umbilicus is common in black infants. Umbilicus should be a bluish white color. Cutis navel (umbilical cord projecting) and granulation tissue in navel are normal. Two arteries and one vein should be apparent. Umbilicus begins drying 1 to 2 hours after birth, blackens by 3 to 5 days, sloughs off by 7 to 9 days. There should be no bleeding.

b. *Deviations:* The following conditions are abnormal findings: umbilical hernia, patent urachus (congenital malformation), omphalocele (congenital hernia), gastroschisis, redness or exudate around cord (infection), yellow discoloration (hemolytic disease, meconium staining), and a single umbilical artery (congenital anomalies).

c. *Evaluation of deviations:* Measure an umbilical hernia by palpating the opening and record. It should close by 1 year of age. Instruct the parents on cord care and hygiene.

d. *Action:* Notify the health care provider from the client's home if a deviation is suspected or apparent.

32. Liver

a. *Standard WNL:* The liver should be 1 to 2 cm below the right costal margin.

b. *Deviations:* An enlarged liver (sepsis, erythroblastosis) requires further evaluation.

c. *Evaluation of deviations:* Note and record size, consistency, and tenderness.

d. *Action:* Notify the health care provider from the client's home if a deviation is suspected or apparent.

33. Spleen

a. *Standards WNL:* The tip should be under the left costal margin. Posterior flank should be firm, oval mass, not enlarged, less commonly palpable.

b. *Deviations:* Enlarged spleen (trauma) or displaced kidney (Wilms' tumor, neuroblastoma, polycryptic kidney, agenesis) are not within normal limits.

c. *Evaluation of deviations:* Assess hydration, voids, other signs and symptoms of infection, kidney failure.

d. *Action:* Notify the health care provider from the client's home if a deviation is suspected or apparent.

34. Auscultation and percussion

    a. *Standards WNL:* Soft bowel sounds may be heard shortly after birth, every 10 to 30 seconds. Normal peristalsis. The abdomen has a tympanic sound except over the liver and spleen (dull sound).

    b. *Deviations:* Bowel sounds in chest (diaphragmatic hernia), an absence of bowel sounds, or hyperperistalsis (intestinal obstruction) are all abnormal findings. Increased dull sound (mass or organomegaly) also is abnormal.

    c. *Evaluation of deviations:* Assess respiratory status; history of bowel movement. Assess for other signs of dehydration or infection. Examine the abdomen thoroughly by light and deep palpation.

    d. *Action:* Notify the health care provider of suspicion and assessment from the client's home.

35. Femoral pulses

    a. *Standards WNL:* Femoral pulses should be palpable, equal, and bilateral.

    b. *Deviations:* Absent or diminished femoral pulses (coarctation of aorta) are not within normal limits.

    c. *Evaluation of deviations:* Evaluate cardiopulmonary status.

    d. *Action:* Notify the health care provider of suspicion and assessment from the client's home.

36. Inguinal area

    a. *Standards WNL:* There should be no bulges along inguinal area and no inguinal lymph nodes felt.

    b. *Deviations:* Inguinal hernia.

    c. *Evaluation of deviations:* Determine if the health care provider is aware of the deviation. Future instruction may be necessary.

    d. *Action:* Call the health care provider with your findings from the client's home unless the parent indicates the provider is already aware of the deviation.

37. Bladder

    a. *Standards WNL:* The bladder percusses 1 to 4 cm above symphysis pubis. It will be emptied about 3 hours after birth, if not at the time of birth. Urine is nonoffensive, with a mild odor.

    b. *Deviations:* Foul odor (infection) and failure to void within 24 hours after birth should be investigated.

    c. *Evaluation of deviations:* Assess hydration, common signs and symptoms of infection, and feeding history.

    d. *Action:* Notify the health care provider from the client's home to report the deviation.

38. Genitals

    a. *Standards WNL:* Gender should be clearly delineated.

    b. *Deviations:* Ambiguous genitals are an abnormal finding.

    c. *Evaluation of deviations:* Review the birth history and the follow-up plan of health care provider.

    d. *Action:* Call the health care provider from the client's home if no follow-up plan has been implemented.

39. Male penis

    a. *Standards WNL:* The penis should be slender in appearance, 2.5 cm long, 1 cm wide at birth. The normal urinary orifice, the urethral meatus, is at the tip of the penis. The urethral opening should be noninflamed. The foreskin adheres to glans, and prepuce can be retracted beyond the urethral opening. Uncircumcised foreskin should be tight after 2 to 3 months. Circumcised. Erectile tissue present.

    b. *Deviations:* Micropenis (congenital anomaly); meatal atresia, hypospadius, epispadius; urethritis (infection); ulceration of meatal opening, infection, inflammation; phimosis, if still tight after 3 months; no foreskin remaining on penis after circumcision are all abnormal findings.

    c. *Evaluation of deviations:* For meatal atresia, observe and record voiding history. For urethritis, palpate for enlarged inguinal lymph nodes and record painful micturition. If meatal opening is ulcerated, evaluate whether the ulcer is due to diaper rash or not. Counsel regarding care. Assess for signs and symptoms of infection. In cases of circumcision, teach parents how to care for circumcision. Teach parents not to retract foreskin of uncircumcised male until told to by health care provider.

    d. *Action:* Report any deviations to the health care provider. Collaborate with the health care provider in the presence of an abnormality.

40. Scrotum

    a. *Standards WNL:* Skin will be loose and hanging or tight and small, and extensive rugae will be present. Scrotum should be of normal size. Scrotal discoloration is common in a breech delivery. Skin should be a normal skin color.

    b. *Deviations:* Large scrotum containing fluid (hydrocele) and red, shiny scrotal skin (orchitis) are abnormal findings.

    c. *Evaluation of deviations:* For hydrocele, shine a light through scrotum (transilluminate) to verify diagnosis. For orchitis, assess for blood supply and tenderness or pain.

    d. *Action:* Notify the health care provider from the client's home of any suspected deviation or problem.

41. Testes

    a. *Standards WNL:* Testes will be descended at birth, and are not consistently found in scrotum. Testes should be 1.5 to 2 cm at birth.

    b. *Deviations:* Undescended testes (cryptorchidism), enlarged testes (tumor), and small testes (Klinefelter's syndrome or adrenal hyperplasia) require further examination.

    c. *Evaluation of deviations:* For cryptorchidism, if the testes cannot be felt in the scrotum, gently palpate femoral inguinal, perineal, and abdominal areas for presence.

    d. *Action:* Notify the health care provider from the client's home of any suspected deviation. Refer and collaborate with the health care provider for further diagnostic studies.

42. Female mons

    a. *Standards WNL:* The female mons should be a normal skin color. The area is pigmented in dark-skinned races. Labia majora cover labia minora, symmetrical size appropriate for gestational age.

    b. *Deviations:* Hematoma and lesions are abnormalities.

    c. *Evaluation of deviations:* Evaluate recent trauma.

    d. *Action:* Notify the health care provider from the client's home of any suspected deviation.

43. Clitoris
    a. *Standard WNL:* The clitoris is normally large in a newborn. Edema and bruising may occur in a breech delivery.
    b. *Deviations:* Hypertrophy (in size; hermaphrodism) is not within normal limits.
    c. *Evaluation of deviations:* Determine if the health care provider is aware of the deviation.
    d. *Action:* Notify the health care provider of your findings.

44. Vagina
    a. *Standards WNL:* Urinary meatus and vaginal orifice are visible (0.5 cm circumference). Vaginal tag or hymenal tag is present, which disappears in a few weeks. There may also be discharge or smegma under labia. Bloody or mucoid discharge is normal as well.
    b. *Deviations:* Inflammation, erythema, and discharge may indicate urethritis. Congenital absence of vagina is another possible problem. A foul-smelling discharge could mean infection. Excessive vaginal bleeding requires evaluation.
    c. *Evaluation of deviations:* If urethritis is suspected, assess for signs and symptoms of infection. Refer any congenital defects to the health care provider. If a discharge is present, collect data and further evaluate the reason for the discharge.
    d. *Action:* Notify the health care provider from the client's home of any suspected deviation.

CHAPTER 3

Invasive Procedures

As part of a comprehensive maternal–child home care program, it is frequently necessary for the nurse to perform invasive procedures. These procedures can be as routine as a follow-up newborn metabolic screening specimen as required by the pediatric provider and the state in which the baby is born. Home care providers should familiarize themselves with the individual laws of their state regarding newborn metabolic screening.

The collection of blood specimens from either the mother or infant may be necessary for a variety of reasons, with blood being drawn by venipuncture or heelstick/fingerstick depending on the type of tests requested. For example, it may be necessary to draw blood specimens in the home to check a newborn's bilirubin level. In the newborn, bilirubin levels do not peak until the third or fourth postpartum day, and most healthy newborns delivered vaginally in this country are discharged within 24 to 48 hours following delivery. Home phototherapy with serial bilirubin levels is today's standard of care for uncomplicated hyperbilirubinemia. Home care providers must also be prepared to test blood sugar in a symptomatic infant or a diabetic mother in case of physician orders. All home care providers should familiarize themselves with laboratory requirements for specimen tube collection, storage, labeling, and delivery time requirements after collection.

The home care nurse may also be called upon to initiate intravenous therapy—for example, to complete a course of antibiotics. This is seen as a safe alternative to hospitalization for those responding to treatment, reducing further risks to the client from nosocomial infection. Increasingly such therapy is becoming a standard of care for both postpartum women and newborns.

Of course, at all times, nurses performing any invasive procedure involving blood should adhere to strict aseptic technique and standard precautions to protect their families and themselves. Procedures regarding the prevention of infection in the home are included in later chapters.

COLLECTION AND RECORDING OF BLOOD SPECIMENS FOR METABOLIC SCREENING

POLICY: A blood specimen for metabolic screening will be obtained from the infant's heel.

PURPOSE: The specimen will be obtained to fulfill state requirements for metabolic screening tests.

PROCEDURE:

1. The agency will verify the need for a metabolic screen with the pediatric care provider for babies discharged 24 hours after birth.
2. The nurse assigned to visit the infant will be responsible for filling in the following information on the screening form.
   a. Name
   b. Address
   c. Date and time of birth
   d. Facility of birth
   e. Physician
   f. Insurance company
   g. Sex, race, birth weight (in grams)
   h. Specimen purpose code
   i. County of residence
   j. Specimen date and time
3. The metabolic specimen is to be collected using the procedure for heel stick. All four circles on both sides of paper are to be completely filled with blood. (When done correctly, blood will seep through front to back.)
4. On the clinical record, document the metabolic screen done and the name of the health care provider giving the order.
5. The specimen must dry thoroughly in the dark for 4 hours before being placed in a wax envelope. (For drying in the dark, a shoe box is suggested.)
6. All completed specimens are to be mailed to the agency on the same day as drawn, or as soon as the specimen has dried adequately.
7. The agency will send copies of the physician's portion of the form to the physician when secured from the laboratory.
8. If a repeat screening is necessary, the pediatric care provider must be contacted for the order and repeat test must be recorded in the metabolic screening book alongside the original. The repeat metabolic screening lab number and date must be recorded.

9. The agency will send the specimen to the state laboratory.
10. The results will be posted in the metabolic screening tracking log.
11. Abnormal levels will be immediately reported to the pediatric care provider.

BLOOD SAMPLE COLLECTION BY HEEL OR FINGER STICK

POLICY:

- A blood sample will be drawn per order.
- Lab results must be noted and reported to the pediatric health care provider to determine if follow-up treatment is necessary.

PURPOSE: Blood will be drawn obtain an acceptable serum sample to be transported to the laboratory for testing.

EQUIPMENT:

1. Alcohol swabs
2. Foot/finger warmer (a warm wash cloth or disposable diaper may also be used.)
3. Sterile lancet
4. Appropriate collection tube (check with the lab performing the test)
5. Band-aid
6. 2 × 2 gauze square
7. Vaseline (optional)
8. Labels
9. Clean gloves

PROCEDURE:

1. You must first receive a referral from the office.
2. Contact the parents by phone to arrange the time of the visit.
3. Explain to the parents that you are going to take a small amount of blood from their child and that they may leave the room if they wish.
4. Expose the infant's foot.
5. Wrap the heel in the foot warmer and allow adequate time for the heel to warm (3 to 5 minutes).
6. Place the infant on a flat surface where he or she will be safe from falling.
7. Put on clean gloves.
8. Remove the warmer and select the puncture site. Cleanse with the site with an alcohol swab. (Optional: Dab on a thin layer of Vaseline.)

9. Puncture the skin with a sterile lancet.

10. Wipe away the first drop of blood with a sterile 2 × 2 gauze pad.

11. If using a microtainer, follow these steps:
    a. Hold the microtainer tube with the Flo Top collector at an angle below horizontal with the vent hole in an upward position.
    b. Touch the tip of the Flo Top collector to the underside of the drop of blood. Blood will flow freely through the Flo Top collector.
    c. Upon termination of the collecting procedure, wipe the wound dry and cover with a Band-aid.
    d. Twist off the Flo Top collector from the tube and discard.
    e. Put a plug securely in the tube opening and label the tube with the infant's name.

12. Inform the parents that you are going to transport the blood sample to the hospital, that the home care agency office will call them with the results, and that their pediatric care provider will also be notified.

13. Call the office with your report of the assessment and the lab drop-off time.

14. Take the blood sample directly to the lab. Protect specimens from sunlight by placing them in a thick padded envelope.

15. Provide the lab with the necessary patient information and request that they call the home care agency office as well as the pediatric care provider's office with the results.

RECOMMENDATIONS FOR SKIN PUNCTURES IN NEWBORNS:

1. Perform heel punctures on the most medial or most lateral portion of the plantar surface of the foot.

2. Puncture no deeper than 2.4 mm.

3. Do not perform punctures on the posterior curvature of the heel.

4. Do not puncture through previous sites that may be infected.

5. For finger stick, use most lateral portions of the palmar side of the third or fourth fingertips.

POLICY AND PROCEDURE: PERIPHERAL VENIPUNCTURE AND BLOOD DRAW

POLICY: The nurse will properly draw blood via peripheral venipuncture per orders.

PURPOSE: A venous blood sample is obtained for prescribed laboratory studies to establish and maintain the proper mode of treatment.

EQUIPMENT:

1. Blood tube container if not using butterfly device
2. Tubes
3. Needles
4. Tourniquet or rubber band
5. Alcohol swabs
6. Povidone–iodine swabs
7. Cotton ball or 2 × 2 sterile gauze square
8. Band-aid
9. Sharps container
10. Latex gloves

PROCEDURE:

1. Explain the procedure to the patient and the parent or caregiver.
2. Assemble all necessary equipment.
3. Wash your hands thoroughly per procedure and put on latex gloves.
4. Assess the status of the upper extremities for a venipuncture site. After a site has been selected, apply a tourniquet or rubber band. The tourniquet or rubber band should be tight enough to trap venous blood but not interfere with arterial flow. If a radial pulse cannot be palpated, the tourniquet or rubber band is too tight.
5. Clean the area with a povidone–iodine swab and/or alcohol–iodine swab and allow to dry.
6. Connect the needle to the blood tube container if not using butterfly device and then place the desired blood tube into the container.

7. Stretch the skin below the vein by holding it firmly with your thumb so the skin is held taut. This will prevent the vein from rolling away from the needle. Perform venipuncture with the needle bevel up. Enter the skin at approximately a 30° angle. Once the needle is through the skin, decrease the angle by lowering the needle hub nearly flush with the skin, and continue inserting with a straight, forward motion. Frequently you will feel a sensation of "release" when you enter the vein.
8. Withdraw the appropriate amount of blood, changing blood tubes if necessary.
9. Remove the tourniquet or rubber band.
10. Remove the needle and apply pressure to the site with a 2 × 2 sterile gauze square. After the bleeding stops, apply a Band-aid. Discard all used sharps and materials in sharps container.
11. Document the procedure on the nursing progress notes.
12. Label the tubes of blood with the patient's name, date, time, and nurse's initials.
13. Notify the case manager of where the blood specimen is being processed.

GUIDE FOR BLOOD TUBE COLLECTION:

1. Red tube: Nonpreserved, plasma and cells separate; electrolytes, chemistries
2. Grey tube: Fasting blood sugar, 2-hour postprandal and random blood sugars
3. Blue tube: Prothrombin time, partial thromboplastin time
4. Purple tube: Complete blood cell count, hemoglobin, hematocrit
5. Green tube: Carbon dioxide content, electrolytes
6. Navy blue tube: Trace elements

NOTES:

1. Different tubes have different preservatives.
2. Preservative-containing tubes should be filled first and gently rotated.
3. Ideally, tubes should be filled to capacity to have proper mix of blood and preservative.
4. Verify tube preference with the local laboratory, because some laboratories may use different colored tubes.
5. Store blood samples in a cool, dry place until they can be taken to the appropriate laboratory.

POLICY AND PROCEDURE: PERIPHERAL VENIPUNCTURE TO INSERT A CATHETER

POLICY: The nurse will maintain the patency of the peripheral line for infusion therapy, as prescribed.

PURPOSE: Maintenance of peripheral patency will permit the prescribed administration of fluids and medication on a continuous or intermittent basis.

EQUIPMENT:

1. Tape (clear tape on babies under 3 years old). Nonallergic tape should be used with excoriated skin.
2. Intravenous cannula as appropriate
3. Sharps container
4. Normal saline
5. Latex gloves
6. Heparinized saline concentration
7. Transparent dressing
8. Injection cap
9. Alcohol swabs
10. Povidone–iodine swabs

FREQUENCY: Intravenous site rotation should occur every 3 days, or more often as needed for phlebitis, thrombosis, infiltration, infection, or other problems (unless otherwise ordered by health care provider).

PROCEDURE:

1. Explain the procedure to the parent or caregiver.
2. Prepare a clean work surface.
3. Organize the supplies needed.
4. Wash your hands (following handwashing procedure) and put on latex gloves.
5. Select IV cannulas.
   a. Butterflies
      1) 23- and 21-gauge butterflies are most frequently used.
      2) For difficult venous access, a 27- or 25-gauge butterfly may be used.

b. Catheters

1) Sizes range from 14- to 24-gauge catheters. The gauge of the needle depends on the newborn's needs.

2) Catheters are used over butterflies in the following instances:

(a) When infusing a drug or solution that is very irritating to the vein.

(b) For infusion via pump.

6. Select insertion site.

a. Examine all extremities for venous access.

b. Begin examining distally and work proximally to the newborn.

c. Only superficial veins are to be used. Veins in the leg and above the ankle are prominent in premature newborns and should not be used due to circulatory compromise of the foot.

d. Contraindications of placement are listed below.

1) Infection, osteomyelitis, and cellulitis—do not use affected extremity.

2) Vasospasm secondary to deep lines with discoloration of an extremity—do not use the affected extremity.

e. Prepare the site.

1) Using a circular motion, cleanse first with alcohol wipes, then with a povidone–iodine swab.

2) Allow to dry for 20 seconds.

f. Insert cannula.

1) Apply a tourniquet to dilate the vein.

2) Put on latex gloves.

3) The site may be numbed with 0.1 or 0.2 ml of normal saline intradermally, using a 27- or 26-gauge needle (optional).

4) Hold the catheter comfortably and firmly for insertion and secure the vein below the insertion site with the other hand.

5) Insert the needle, bevel up, through the skin parallel to the vein, until blood return is achieved. Thread cannula until the hub is proximal to the skin surface. ***Note:*** Pre-sticking with a 21- or 22-gauge needle for a 22- or 24-gauge catheter may be done to ease insertion (optional).

6) No more than three attempts may be made by one nurse. Table 3-1 shows some common problems that can arise and solutions for these problems.

7) Secure the cannula in place with tape.

(a) Do not apply tape too tightly because pressure sores may occur, especially under the hub of the catheter.

(b) Do not place tape directly over the site.

(c) Apply povidone–iodine ointment to all catheters and a transparent dressing over the insertion site.

8) Remove the tourniquet and stylet.

9) Connect either intravenous tubing or an injection cap (heparin lock) into the cannula and secure.
   (a) For an injection cap (heparin lock), flush with heparin and check for patency by aspirating for blood return and observe for signs/symptoms of infiltration.
   (b) In giving a medication dose, the heparin lock is flushed with 0.3 ml of normal saline. Administer the medication, then 0.3 ml of normal saline flush after the medication dose, then the heparin flush (1 ml normal saline/10 units of heparin solution).
   (c) Minimum flushing of injection cap (heparin lock) is once per day when not in use.
10) Document the insertion site, gauge of catheter, date and time of insertion, nurse's initials, and any complications of the procedure. This should be noted on the nursing progress notes.
11) Inform the and parent or caregiver of signs and symptoms of complications and rationale and performance of this procedure as appropriate.
12) Discard all used materials in sharps container.

TABLE 3-1
Guidelines for Problematic Patient Conditions

Patient Condition	Effect on Patient	Guidelines
Shock; sepsis, hypotension	Poor perfusion, vasoconstriction, difficult to locate veins	1. Flush fluid through needle 2. Use different tourniquet tensions or blood pressure cuff techniques 3. Expect no blood return 4. Inserter rarely feels needle enter the vein 5. Soaks may help but are not very effective 6. Squeeze distally and proximally to site at the same time to pump up the vein
Increased temp., febrile	Dilated veins	1. May not get blood return 2. Usually easier to find veins
Decreased body temperature due to: cold environment, use of cooling mattress, use of multiple swabs with alcohol on babies.	Vasoconstriction	1. Apply warm soaks over a large area 2. Wrap with blanket and wait 30 minutes 3. Use warmer bed if available 4. Use different tourniquet tensions or blood pressure cuff techniques 5. Expect minimal blood return
Fear vasoconstriction	Fight or flight	1. Control breathing; insert needle when patient is exhaling 2. Have patient blow out candles or shout Ouch!
Jaundice or bililights (phototherapy), low platelets	Fragile veins	1. Apply low tourniquet tension 2. Insert needle into vein slowly and advance gently 3. Remove tourniquet rapidly
Malnutrition: poor skin turgor, poor muscle tone	Large, unstabilized veins	1. Exaggerate skin tension 2. Insert whole unit in the vein before advancing the catheter
Flaccidity: very poor muscle tone, loose skin	Rolling veins not visible or palpable	1. Rely on anatomy 2. Exaggerate skin tension 3. Using the veins of the feet is usually easier
Obesity	Veins not visible	1. Digital veins are often visible 2. Rely on anatomy
Edema	Veins not visible	1. Press out fluid 2. Test for refill 3. Insert needle far enough into the vein so that returning fluid will not push the needle out
Long-term therapy	Damaged veins; many collateral veins	1. Use any necessary guidelines

POLICY AND PROCEDURE: PERIPHERAL LINE AND HEPARIN LOCK APPLICATION

POLICY: The nurse will insert and maintain heparin lock patency as prescribed.

PURPOSE: The nurse will maintain an intravenous line via a heparin lock for patients requiring venous access for medication. Allow the patient freedom of mobility.

PROCEDURE:

1. Follow nursing procedure for peripheral venipuncture, assessment of site, insertion of catheter, and taping of site.
2. Flush heparin lock with 0.5 to 1 ml of heparin flush solution (1 ml normal saline/10 units heparin solution) at the time of insertion of the heparin lock and after each dose of medication.
3. In giving the medication dose, the heparin lock is flushed with 0.3 ml of normal saline. Administer the medication, then 0.3 ml of normal saline flush after the medication dose, then the heparin flush (1 ml normal saline/10 units of heparin solution).
4. Assess the intravenous site at the time of flushing for infiltration, phlebitis, and/or leaking.
5. Document on the Nursing Medication Sheet and Nursing Progress Notes the following information.
    a. Date and time heparin lock was started
    b. Date and time site was changed
    c. Gauge of intravenous needle
    d. Medication administered
    e. Assessment of site
6. Properly discard all materials in sharps container.
7. Educate family member or caregiver in the procedure for applying pressure to the site if the heparin lock should become dislodged.

POLICY AND PROCEDURE: PERIPHERAL INTRAVENOUS COMPLICATIONS

POLICY: The nurse should be able to recognize signs and symptoms of peripheral intravenous therapy complications.

PURPOSE: Expedient recognition will allow the nurse to apply the appropriate intervention for complications of intravenous therapy.

PROCEDURE:

1. Phlebitis: Inflammation of the walls of the vein.
   a. *Cause:* Direct injury/trauma to the vein from intravenous injections, indwelling catheters, overuse of a vein, infusion of an irritating solution, use of a large-bore cannula, long-term cannula placement, or extension of an infection into the tissue surrounding the vessel.
   b. *Symptoms:* Venous distention, edema, local heat, erythema, induration, or pain at the site of cannula placement and along the course of the affected vein.
   c. *Intervention:* Identify and document the symptoms. Change the IV site. Apply cold compresses for 24 hours, with moist heat thereafter to stimulate circulation and promote absorption. Continue observation for elevated temperature, purulence, pain, erythema, or local heat at the identified site. Notify the health care provider of the intervention and obtain further prescribed orders.
2. Thrombosis: Clot formation in the cannula or vessel that occludes flow through the catheter or vessel.
   a. *Cause:* Usually caused by stasis of blood in catheter by patient position or neglectful heparinization of the catheter.
   b. *Symptoms:* Inability to flush catheter, erythema, inflammation, induration of insertion site.
   c. *Intervention:* Discontinue peripheral intravenous line according to procedure. Notify the health care provider and proceed as prescribed.
3. Infiltration: Accumulation of fluid in tissue surrounding intravenous cannula.
   a. *Cause:* Dislocation of cannula or loss of vessel integrity.
   b. *Symptoms:* Edema, skin blanching, pain, decreased temperature of skin at the site as well as slowing or cessation of intravenous fluid not associated with mechanical or tubing problems. ***Note:*** A blood return may still be present with infiltration.
   c. *Intervention:* Discontinue infusion and cannula. Apply warm compresses to site of infiltrate to increase fluid absorption. Notify health care provider and proceed as prescribed.
4. Embolism: Obstruction of a blood vessel by a blood clot or a foreign substance.
   a. *Cause:* Most common cause is dislodging of a thrombus into systemic circulation.
   b. *Symptoms:* Ischemia, hypotension, dyspnea, cyanosis, tachycardia, peripheral numbness, tingling, and loss of consciousness.

   c. *Intervention:* Call health care provider immediately and initiate emergency procedure, as should be stated in the policies of all providers of this service. ***Note:*** If a catheter fragment has entered the systemic circulation, immediately apply firm pressure (proximal manual tourniquet) to contain the fragment.

5. Infection: Intravenous site that has been invaded by pathogenic organisms producing deleterious effects locally and systemically.
   a. *Cause:* Poor aseptic technique, contamination of the catheter and/or solution, and intrinsic factors (immunosuppression, steroid therapy, or malnutrition)
   b. *Symptoms:* Fever, chills, tachycardia, erythema, inflammation, purulence, pain, and localized heat from insertion site
   c. *Intervention:* Prevent infection by inspecting solution and supplies for contamination. Properly review and practice aseptic techniques. Notify health care provider of signs and symptoms and proceed with prescribed orders.

TEACHING CAREGIVERS AND PATIENTS:

1. For all of the complications described above, the caregivers and patients are to be educated concerning the following information.
   a. The condition and the definition of the condition
   b. Symptomatology
   c. Proper interventions
2. All teaching by the infusion nurse should be documented and reviewed at each visit.

POLICY AND PROCEDURE: DISCONTINUATION OF PERIPHERAL INTRAVENOUS CATHETER

POLICY: The nurse will discontinue the peripheral intravenous catheter properly when prescribed.

PURPOSE: An intravenous cannula will be removed when intravenous access is no longer prescribed, when site rotation is necessary, or when complications exist.

PROCEDURE:

1. Place gauze over the site of the cannula insertion and withdraw cannula.
2. Hold the gauze in place with slight pressure being applied for 2 to 3 minutes.
3. Check the site for continued bleeding. ***Note:*** If bleeding continues, apply pressure or pressure dressing.
4. If there is no bleeding, apply a bandage or gauze with tape.
5. Discard all materials in sharps container.
6. Document on the Nursing Progress Notes the time, date, and assessment of the site after discontinuation.

CHAPTER 4

Standard Program for High-Risk Newborn Home Visiting Follow-Up

This program was developed after 6 years of research in problems related to newborn mortality. The home health agency that developed this program implemented it in 1992 in its service area that included many neighborhoods in Philadelphia with high infant mortality rates. The program was fully implemented in 1993, using strategies proven effective by home health visiting programs for high-risk infants throughout North America and abroad.

This program is designed to provide home visiting follow-up to newborns identified as high risk, either at the time of hospital discharge or at a newborn home visit made shortly after the newborn is discharged from the hospital and continues throughout the infant's first year of life.

HIGH-RISK NEWBORN FOLLOW-UP PROGRAM

Criteria for Admission

The criteria for admission to the program incorporate those risk factors associated with a high incidence of infant mortality and morbidity. Admission criteria for program inclusion are as follow:

1. The infant's birth weight is 1500 grams or less.
2. The infant is born to a mother who is 17 years old or younger.
3. The infant is born to a mother who received no prenatal care, had less than 4 prenatal visits, or began prenatal care in the third trimester.
4. The newborn or mother has a positive urine drug screen or there is maternal drug or alcohol abuse.
5. The newborn or mother is infected with HIV.
6. Acceptance into the program has been deemed medically necessary by the pediatric care provider.

Initial Newborn Home Visit

1. The first home visit will be completed within 24–72 hours of discharge as determined by medical condition at hospital discharge.
2. The following paperwork is to be completed and submitted to the office:
   a. Consent for Treatment, Release of Information, Assignment of Benefits, Notice of Client Rights. Copies of these forms should also be provided to the client.
   b. Newborn Universal Home Assessment Tool
   c. Plan of Care
   d. Clinical Time Log/Encounter Form

Cases Eligible for the High-Risk Newborn Follow-up Program

1. Newborns identified as high risk at the time of the newborn referral or newborn visit are eligible for the program.
2. A Comprehensive Initial Evaluation Visit is necessary and entails the following:
   a. A Comprehensive Evaluation Visit will be scheduled within one week of the first newborn home visit for those infants admitted to the High-Risk Newborn Home Visiting program. It is recommended that all newborns receive access to at least one visit in order to assure universal home risk assessment. Not all newborns receiving access to universal home risk assessment will be admitted to the High-Risk Newborn Home Visiting Follow-Up Program. For those newborns fitting the admission criteria, this will be the second visit. Newborns not fitting the admission criteria may be discharged or may receive a home visit plan that does not necessitate a year-long follow-up program. The

nurse should complete the Initial Evaluation Form and the Home Needs Assessment Tool (found in the Appendix) as part of this visit, incorporating information from the Newborn Universal Home Assessment Tool completed at the first home visit.

b. Newborns will be seen according to an individualized Plan of Care established by the pediatric care provider for the program. The Plans of Care must be reevaluated every 62 days throughout the infant's first year of life.

c. The following paperwork is to be completed and submitted to the office.

1) Consent for Treatment, Release of Information, Assignment of Benefits, Notice of Client Rights. Copies of these forms should also be provided to the client.

2) Initial Evaluation Form

3) Home Needs Assessment Form

4) Plan of Care for first 62 days

5) Clinical Time Log/Encounter Form

3. Follow-up visits

a. Follow-up visits will be performed according to the Standard Plans of Care or any addenda ordered by the pediatric care provider.

b. The following paperwork is to be completed and submitted to the office:

1) Nursing Plan of Care and Progress Record

2) Clinical Time Log/Encounter Form

3) Revised Plan of Treatment every 62 days

4. Deviations from standard protocol
Every attempt should be made to see newborns according to the visit frequency established in the Plan of Care. If this does not occur, an addendum to the Plan of Treatment must be completed by the nurse and forwarded to the pediatric care provider for his or her signature.

5. The nurse should know the proper person to contact when a problem arises.

a. The clinical administrator should be contacted for any patient care or health status questions, or before referrals to a child protective agency.

b. The business manager should be contacted for any questions or concerns regarding the health insurance status of the client. He or she should be notified immediately of any changes in health insurance to ensure reimbursement for all nursing visits.

c. The administrative secretary should be contacted regarding any questions or changes to the client visit schedule or when a client requires assistance in accessing community resources.

d. The pediatric care provider should be notified of any abnormalities or deteriorations of health status noted at the time of the client visit. If the nurse is unsure whether or not to notify the pediatric care provider, the clinical administrator should be consulted.

Discharge Criteria

Newborns will be discharged from the program for any of the following reasons:

1. Insurance changed or denied: The newborn's insurance has changed to a payor who does not reimburse for the program or prior authorization of the services has been denied.

2. Unable to locate: After repeated attempts, the newborn cannot be located.
3. Refused visits: The caregiver has refused to continue visits for the newborn.
4. Noncompliance
5. Goals met: The newborn has reached the first birthday and achieved the goals stated in the Plan of Care.
6. Rehospitalized: The newborn has been admitted to the hospital for two weeks or longer.
7. Moved out of service area: The newborn's family has moved outside of the agency's service area.
8. Transferred: The newborn has been transferred to the care of another home health agency.
9. Placed or adopted: The newborn has been placed in foster care or adopted.
10. Expired

Data Collection

Information regarding the newborn referrals and their disposition is collected and reported on a monthly and quarterly basis. A program summary should be prepared annually and presented to the professional advisory committee. Data collection forms can be found in the Appendix.

The number of newborns admitted to the home care program should correspond to the geographic area's newborn mortality rate (that is, if the agency visits a geographic area with a newborn mortality rate of 15%, the number admitted to high-risk newborn home care identified through universal screening should reflect a similar percentage).

High-Risk Home Visiting Follow-up Plan

Box 3-1 is an actual schedule of visits and what is entailed at each visit. Visits may be done by a nurse–social worker team or by the nurse alone (in this case the nurse must have community resource experience). For this reason, some visits will mention a social worker's presence.

BOX 3-1: HOME VISIT SCHEDULE

Content of Visit	Timing of Home Visit	Key Points to Evaluate (No Complications)	Key Points to Evaluate (Special Care Infants)
The nurse should assess, observe, and evaluate the medical, psychosocial, and developmental status of the mother and newborn. Plan and provide interventions for identified problems. Assess client's educational needs and skills to perform technical care. Provide guidance in caregiver skills involving feeding, nutrition, breastfeeding support, normal and abnormal behavior development needs, and danger signs. Assist with coordination of equipment, medical supplies, prescriptions, emergency plan, and WIC screens.	24–72 hours after discharge for maternal–newborn clients without delivery/postpartum/neonatal problems. 24 hours after discharge for maternal–newborn clients with delivery/postpartum/neonatal complications.	At discharge, the nurse should perform the following tasks. 1. Identify pediatric provider. 2. Assess medical needs. 3. Intervene if there are any medical problems. 4. Determine social/support needs. 5. Identify the necessary medical equipment and supplies. 6. Schedule appointments: WIC (if eligible), pediatric provider, insurance. 7. Assist with prescription problems. 8. Identify special needs.	At discharge, the nurse should perform the following tasks. 1. Identify pediatric provider. 2. Assess medical needs. 3. Intervene if there are any medical problems. 4. Determined social/support needs. 5. Identify the necessary medical equipment and supplies. 6. Schedule appointments: WIC (if eligible), pediatric provider, insurance. 7. Assist with prescription problems. 8. Identify special needs.
The nurse or social worker should assess, observe, evaluate, and plan and provide interventions for identified problems. An individual needs-based plan should be developed.	1 week after discharge	1. The infant's appointment with the pediatric provider should be made. 2. Assess growth and development, and physical status. 3. Assist in scheduling WIC appointment, if eligible. 4. Identify appointments not made and help facilitate appointments. 5. Identify individual social problems. Facilitate resolution. 6. Assess the need for welfare, family planning, and pediatric provider. 7. Assist with access to public or low cost child health insurance, if needed.	1. The infant's appointment with the pediatric provider should be made. 2. Assess growth and development, and physical status. 3. Assist in scheduling WIC appointment, if eligible. 4. Identify appointments not made and help facilitate appointments. 5. Identify individual social problems. Facilitate resolution. 6. Assess the need for welfare, family planning, and pediatric provider. 7. Assist with access to public or low cost child health insurance, if needed. 8. Infant high risk appointment. 9. Check medical supplies and medicinal needs.

The nurse should assess, observe, and evaluate the medical, psychosocial, and developmental status. Plan and provide interventions for identified problems. Monitor health and resolution of identified problems. Provide teaching based on appropriate feeding, newborn weight gain, development, parenting, infant behaviors, maternal feelings, safety, car seats, bath safety, and hygiene.	Visits weekly between 2 and 4 weeks	1. Pediatric provider, 2 weeks. 2. Maternal WIC appointment, if eligible, 3 weeks. 3. Pediatric WIC appointment, if eligible, 3 weeks. 4. Assess growth and development.	1. Pediatric provider, 2 weeks. 2. Maternal WIC appointment, if eligible, 3 weeks. 3. Pediatric WIC appointment, if eligible, 3 weeks. 4. Assess growth and development. 5. Assess need for medical supplies, equipment, and prescriptions.
The nurse or social worker should assess, observe, evaluate, and plan and provide interventions for identified problems. Provide direct assistance with identified barriers to healthcare. Monitoring identified problems, appropriate behaviors, developments, and parental attachment. Assure access to health insurance for mother and/or infant and/or budgeting of welfare benefits.	5 weeks after discharge	1. Follow up on insurance coverage if it continues to be a problem. 2. Pediatric provider, 5 weeks. 3. Family planning, 6 weeks. 4. Assess growth and development.	1. Follow up on insurance coverage if it continues to be a problem. 2. Pediatric provider, 5 weeks. 3. Family planning, 6 weeks. 4. Assess growth and development. 5. Assess need for medical supplies, equipment, and prescriptions. 6. Determine if the infant is being followed through a high risk infant hospital program and establish communication with the neonatologist, if the infant is enrolled in this type of program.
The nurse should assess, observe, and evaluate the medical, psychosocial, and developmental status. Plan and provide interventions for identified problems. Monitor the health of the mother and infant. Reinforce and facilitate family planning; instruct about infant weight gain, immunizations, vision, and hearing. Monitor safety, safety hazards, nutrition/feeding, child/day care, the health of the family, dental, vision, hearing, and danger signs. Identify the maternal primary care provider.	8 weeks after discharge	1. Maternal primary provider appointment, 9 weeks. 2. WIC appointment, if eligible, 8 weeks. 3. Pediatric provider appointment, 8-9 weeks (immunizations). 4. Assess growth and development.	1. Maternal primary provider appointment, 9 weeks. 2. WIC appointment, if eligible, 8 weeks. 3. Pediatric provider appointment, 8-9 weeks (immunizations). 4. Assess growth and development. 5. Assess need for medical supplies, equipment, and prescriptions.

(continued)

BOX 3-1: HOME VISIT SCHEDULE (continued)

Content of Visit	Timing of Home Visit	Key Points to Evaluate (No Complications)	Key Points to Evaluate (Special Care Infants)
The nurse should assess, observe, and evaluate the medical, psychosocial, and developmental status. Plan and provide interventions for identified problems. Monitor health status and access to care. Educate parents concerning fire safety, electric, stress, feeding, nutrition, general family safety, poison, hygiene, and allergies. Assess medicinal needs and immunizations.	12–16 weeks after discharge	1. Pediatric provider appointment (immunizations), 3–4 months. 2. Assess growth and development.	1. Pediatric provider appointment (immunizations), 3-4 months. 2. Assess growth and development. 3. Assess need for medical supplies, equipment, and prescriptions.
The nurse should assess, observe, and evaluate the medical, psychosocial, and developmental status. Plan and provide interventions for identified problems. Monitor health status. Provide resources to the mother as desired: education, jobs, day care, Head Start, home safety, environmental, infant behaviors, development, parenting, stress, and immunization status.	16–20 weeks after discharge	1. Pediatric provider appointment, 5 months. 2. WIC appointment, if eligible, 5 months. 3. Assess growth and development.	1. Pediatric provider appointment, 5 months. 2. WIC appointment, if eligible, 5 months. 3. Assess growth and development.
The nurse or social worker should assess, observe, and evaluate the medical, psychosocial, and developmental status. Plan and provide interventions for identified problems. Reassess plan, and determine the need to reassess welfare. Evaluate parenting skills and budgeting.	25–26 weeks	1. Pediatric provider appointment (immunizations), 6 months. 2. WIC appointment, if eligible, 6 and 7 months. 3. Assess growth and development.	1. Pediatric provider appointment (immunizations), 6 months. 2. WIC appointment, if eligible, 6 and 7 months. 3. Return to high risk clinic. 4. Assess growth and development. 5. Assess the need for medical supplies, equipment, and prescriptions.

The nurse will focus on the provision of assessments and interventions which will identify problems requiring early intervention. Evaluate the effectiveness of the nursing service provided each visit. Focus with the family on education, centered on the emotional and developmental needs of the family/infant.	29–30 weeks	1. Pediatric provider appointment (immunizations), 8 months. 2. WIC appointment, if eligible, 8 months. 3. Assess growth and development.	1. Pediatric provider appointment (immunizations), 8 months. 2. WIC appointment, if eligible, 8 months. 3. Assess growth and development. 4. Assess the need for medical supplies, equipment, and prescriptions.
The nurse will assess, observe, and evaluate the medical, psychosocial, and developmental status. Plan and provide interventions for identified problems. Monitor health, hearing, vision, feeding, nutrition, appropriate behaviors, and development. Assess the need for primary care of other family members and public health issues.	35–37 weeks	1. Pediatric provider appointment (immunizations), 10 months. 2. WIC appointments, if eligible, 7–12 months. 3. Assess growth and development.	1. Pediatric provider appointment (immunizations), 10 months. 2. WIC appointments, if eligible, 7–12 months. 3. Assess growth and development. 4. Assess the need for medical supplies, equipment, and prescriptions.
The nurse will assess, observe, and evaluate the medical, psychosocial, and developmental status. Plan and provide interventions for identified problems. Monitor health status of infant/family. Teach home safety, cleaning items, food storage, safety locks, steps, and swimming pools. Reenforce both electric and fire safety. Teach appropriate behaviors for age.	41–43 weeks.	1. Pediatric provider appointment (immunizations), 11 months. 2. WIC appointment, if eligible.	1. Pediatric provider appointment (immunizations), 11 months. 2. WIC appointment, if eligible. 3. Assess growth and development. 4. Assess the need for medical supplies, equipment, and prescriptions.
The nurse will assess, observe, and evaluate the medical, psychosocial, and developmental status. Plan and provide interventions for identified problems. Monitor health status/follow-up of problems, age-appropriate behavior, stress, nutrition, feeding, safety (cribs, furniture, outlets) and follow-up health care plans designed for family. Reinforce healthy environments, immunizations, and discharge to the care of a physician.	43–52 weeks.	1. Pediatric provider appointment (immunizations), 12 months. 2. WIC appointment, if eligible. 3. Assess growth and development.	1. Pediatric provider appointment (immunizations), 12 months. 2. WIC appointment, if eligible. 3. Assess growth and development. 4. Assess the need for medical supplies, equipment, and prescriptions. 5. Return to high risk clinic, if enrolled.

HIGH-RISK FOLLOW-UP OUTCOME MEASURES

GOAL	MEASUREMENT
BIRTH to 2 MONTHS	
Linkage to health care system and PCP (pediatric care provider) identified	Family knows health care provider's name, phone number, and how to make appointment
Newborn home visits	Appointment kept
Initial newborn visit (PCP)	At least 1 newborn visit appointment kept
ER use and rehospitalization minimized	No inappropriate ER visits or preventable hospitalizations
Social/Financial Support	
Health insurance for newborn	Child has health insurance, private or through state
Adequate maternal food	Has access to balanced diet and food stamps
Adequate infant food	Has access to breastfeeding or formula
WIC referral and appointment (if eligible)	WIC appointment kept
Adequate newborn supplies	Has clothing, diapers, bottles and a place for newborn to sleep
Transportation for health care appointments	Identified source of transportation (e.g., car, bus, cab)
Mental health/drug/alcohol counseling	Appointment scheduled and kept
Parenting problems identified and addressed	Teaching initiated; referrals initiated
Newborn Nutrition	
Adequate food	Access to formula; enrolled in WIC
Appropriate weight gain	Weight gain of 4–6 oz per week for full-term newborn and 3–4 oz per week for premature newborn
Other: list specific need	Referral or other problem solving initiated
2–4 MONTHS	
Newborn Nutrition	
Appropriate growth and weight gain	Growth consistent with weight graph
Developmental milestones reached	Documented in home care chart
Appropriate utilization of health care system	Caregiver is compliant with appointments
Appointment for immunizations kept	Immunizations received on schedule
Lead level determined	Lead level known
Enrolled in EPSDT program (if eligible)	Receiving care from EPSDT provider
Social/Financial Support	
Referrals previously initiated in place	Appointments kept
Other: list specific need	
Referral or other problem solving initiated	

(continued)

GOAL	MEASUREMENT
4–6 MONTHS	
Newborn Nutrition	
Appropriate growth and weight gain	Growth consistent with weight graph
Nutritional support and teaching	Documented in home care chart
Transition from formula to baby food begun	Documented in home care chart
Developmental milestones reached	Documented in home care chart
Appropriate utilization of health care system	Caregiver is compliant with appointments
Appointment for immunizations kept	Immunizations received on schedule
Lead level drawn at 6 mos	Lead level known
Social/Financial Support	
Referrals previously initiated in place	Appointments kept
Other: List specific need	Referral or other problem solving initiated
6–8 MONTHS	
Newborn Nutrition	
Appropriate growth and weight gain	Growth consistent with weight graph
Developmental milestones reached	Documented in home care chart
Social/Financial Support	
Any outstanding problems addressed	Documented in home care chart
Other: list specific need	Referral or other problem solving initiated
8–10 MONTHS	
Newborn Nutrition	
Appropriate growth and weight gain	Growth consistent with weight graph
Developmental milestones reached	Documented in home care chart
Appropriate utilization of health care system	Caregiver is compliant with appointments
Lead level drawn by 9 mos	If first lead level known, result was $>10–14$ μg/dl
Social/Financial Support	
Any outstanding problems addressed	Documented in home care chart
Other: list specific need	Referral or other problem solving initiated
10–12 MONTHS	
Newborn Nutrition	
Appropriate growth and weight gain	Growth consistent with weight graph
Developmental milestones reached	Documented in home care chart
Appropriate utilization of health care system	Caregiver is compliant with appointments
Adequately immunized	All first year immunizations received
Lead level drawn by 12 mos	If first lead level known, result was >10 μg/dl
Social/Financial Support	
Any outstanding problems addressed	Documented in home care chart
Other: list specific need	Referral or other problem solving initiated
Discharge planning	Any ongoing needs and sources of support are documented in the home care chart

CHAPTER 5

Specific Protocols Used in Maternal–Newborn Follow-Up

This chapter contains protocols the nurse will find useful in providing maternal–newborn home visiting. The protocols were developed to address some of the most commonly used home care procedures for more complex maternal–child procedures. Included are home phototherapy, apnea monitoring, neonatal abstinence due to drug withdrawal, and intravenous therapy. Maternal protocols include staple removal for women with cesarean deliveries, and wound dehiscence. Although we all wish every delivery resulted in a happy outcome, that is not always possible. Nurses working in maternal–child home health must be prepared to assist families when a positive outcome is not possible. A protocol for a bereavement visit is also included for the nurse's information.

Additional protocols are included to help reduce the risks of infection, for both the family and the nurse. Nurses will find these helpful to use as a standard of practice, and administrators can include this section in the orientation of all new nurses.

HOME CARE PROTOCOL: FIBEROPTIC HOME PHOTOTHERAPY

Phototherapy will be initiated per order in accordance with agency general admission criteria and the criteria below.

Eligibility Requirements

1. The pediatric health care provider must refer the patient to the phototherapy program with a diagnosis of idiopathic neonatal hyperbilirubinemia.
2. The newborn must meet the following criteria:
   a. The newborn's birth weight must be over 2270 grams.
   b. The newborn must be term (37 to 40 weeks).
   c. Apgar scores should be above 7.
   d. Only vigorous, active newborns will be admitted to the program.
   e. The newborn must be feeding without difficulty.
   f. There should be adequate stooling and urination within 24 hours of birth.
   g. The newborn blood levels should be as follows:
      1) Combs test: negative
      2) Rh-sensitization: negative
      3) ABO incompatibility: negative (an ABO incompatibility in which bilirubin level is trending downward will be considered for admission; the infant's hemoglobin level must be known)
      4) Direct bilirubin: <1.5 mg/100 ml
      5) Hematocrit: less than 65%
      6) Total bilirubin level within the previous 6 hours
      7) Maternal and infant blood types must be known.
   h. The history of bilirubin level at various ages should be known (this is a guideline only).
      1) At 24 hours old, below 10 mg/100 ml
      2) At 48 hours old, below 15 mg/100 ml
      3) At 72 hours old or older, below 18 mg/100 ml
3. There should be no educational or language barriers with the parents.
4. The newborn should have an adequate home environment (there should be electricity, heat, and phone).
5. Plan for follow-up bilirubin levels daily or twice daily, depending on the orders.
6. The parents should be aware of their 24-hour monitoring responsibility.

Equipment Needed

1. Home phototherapy blanket unit containing illuminator, fiberoptic cable and panel, and disposable panel covers
2. Thermometer
3. Equipment for drawing blood samples
4. Phototherapy chart packet
   a. Parent information sheet
   b. Consent form/initial evaluation chart
   c. Nursing progress/Plan of Care
   d. Parent's record of phototherapy treatment
   e. Discharge summary
5. Three-prong grounded plug adapter

Procedure

1. Wash your hands and complete the infant assessment.
2. Provide the parents with the parent information sheet and review the family teaching sheet.
3. The illuminator box should be placed only on a hard, flat surface, no more than 4 feet from where the baby will be lying or held. Be sure that the air vent in the rear of the unit is not blocked. Do not put the illuminator next to or on a radiator or heater.
4. Insert the metal collar of the fiberoptic panel completely into the insert of the illuminator. The end of the metal collar of the fiberoptic panel is designed to be even with the end of the insert of the illuminator. Turn the metal collar of the panel clockwise, one quarter-turn, to lock it in place.
5. Plug the illuminator box into an electrical outlet. You will need a three-prong plug (grounded) outlet close by for the electrical cord. A heavy-duty extension cord, such as those used for power tools or appliances, can be used.
6. Insert the panel into a disposable panel cover, ensuring that the light faces the fabric side of the cover, not the plastic side.
7. Place the covered panel around the baby, under his or her arms. Be sure that the fabric side goes against the skin. The lower part of the panel will be on the outside of the baby's diaper. Be sure the diaper is folded down below the baby's navel in front and as far as possible in the back so that as much of the skin as possible is exposed to the light.
8. Using two of the tape tabs provided, fasten the panel in place by affixing the tabs on the plastic side of the cover at the open end close to where you inserted the fiberoptic panel. You should be able to insert two fingers between the panel and the baby's skin if applied properly.

9. You can now place a T-shirt on the baby, and wrap him or her in a blanket or a sleeper. In larger or more active babies, to prevent possible skin irritation under the baby's arms, tuck a little of the baby's T-shirt, blanket, or sleeper into the top of the panel. Doing this will help cushion the infant's armpit area, preventing skin irritation.

10. Turn on the illuminator and start therapy.

11. Inform the parents of the follow-up visit plan.

12. Return for bilirubin draws as per pediatric care provider orders and deliver to the preidentified laboratory.

13. Notify the home care agency office (or the on-call supervisor) of the estimated time the lab report will be available; provide the names and phone numbers of the pediatric care provider and the laboratory.

14. The home care nurse (or the on-call supervisor) is responsible for obtaining the lab result, contacting the pediatric care provider, and coordinating the plan for further orders.

HOME CARE PROTOCOL: APNEA MONITOR

Eligibility Requirements

1. The initial acute treatment has been completed.
2. Laboratory test values are within the normal range.
3. A pneumogram and other pertinent sleep studies have been completed.
4. The newborn is free of infection.
5. The parents have received CPR and monitor training.
6. The newborn is receiving an adequate amount of formula to promote an average weight gain of 15 to 20 grams per 24 hours; this applies to the premature neonate only, because weight gain is not a significant indicator for discharge of the older newborn.
7. The pediatric care provider has been selected.
8. The predischarge assessment in the home has been completed.
9. All of the necessary equipment has been ordered.
10. The patient has been discharged 24 to 48 hours after meeting the discharge criteria.
11. The electric company has been notified of the medical need for power priority.
12. The appropriate utilities have been notified of the need for water, phone, electricity, and heat in cases of economic hardship.
13. An emergency transport plan is in place.

General Nursing and Pediatric Care Provider Treatment Orders

Before discharge of the patient from the hospital, a predischarge evaluation is to be completed. The Home Needs Assessment Tool found in the appendices can be used for this purpose. This evaluation entails the following:

1. Socioeconomic evaluation
2. Laboratory tests
3. Neonatal testing results (if appropriate)
4. Complete physical assessment and history to include the following information:
   a. Birth history and hospital course
   b. Appropriate identifying information
      1) Newborn's name, address, phone number
      2) Parents' names

3) Referring pediatric care provider's name, address, phone number
4) Insurance type and numbers
5) Type of home care, visits, and frequency

c. Medications and dietary/treatment orders
d. Supplies and equipment needed
e. Evaluation of initial visit, establishing long-term and short-term goals
f. Signature of the pediatric nurse and date the predischarge assessment was rendered

5. The schedule of home visits by the monitor company set up to alternate with nursing visits
6. Notification of the electric company of the state of medical priority for any child using medical electrical equipment in case of a power outage
7. Notification of the appropriate utilities of the need for water, phone, electricity, and heat in cases of economic hardship
8. Establishment of an emergency transport plan with the family and the appropriate local transport team

Nursing Assessment Each Visit

The nurse will perform physical assessment and examination to evaluate the following areas:

1. Respiratory: Auscultate the lungs for rate, rhythm, and abnormal breath sounds. Observe the character of respiratory effort (retractions, grunting, or flaring).
2. Metabolic: Assess the patient's temperature and intake.
3. Gastrointestinal: Assess for vomiting, frequent loose stools, and irritation of buttocks. Weigh the newborn, measure girth, and auscultate bowel sounds.
4. Genitourinary: Determine the number of wet diapers per 24 hours.
5. Musculoskeletal: Check muscle tone, vigor of activity, and movement of all extremities.
6. Neurologic: Assess the fontanel, irritability, cry, presence of jitteriness or seizure activity.
7. Determine number of times the alarm has sounded and the reasons why.
8. Cardiovascular: Assess the heart rate, rhythm, presence of murmur, central and peripheral color, and peripheral pulses.

Activity

The child's activity should be limited to in the home and should be appropriate for the child's age and development.

Diet

1. Review the newborn's intake.
2. Formula and volume will be determined by the pediatric care provider.

Education

1. Safety
    a. Review newborn safety; identify and correct hazards in the home.
    b. Review signs of infection, feeding intolerance, and seizures with the parents.
    c. Review the monitor and CPR with the parents; assess their understanding of apnea and what happens if the alarm sounds.
2. Growth and development
    a. Review newborn development and stimulation to promote growth.
    b. Reinforce the need for immunizations and follow-up visits.
3. Drugs: Educate the family concerning the signs and symptoms of adverse reactions to the medications prescribed.
4. Miscellaneous: Inform the parents of available community resources.

HOME CARE PROTOCOL: EDUCATING PARENTS/CAREGIVERS ABOUT DIARRHEA AND NUTRITION

The major complication from gastroenteritis is dehydration and accompanying electrolyte imbalance. Signs of dehydration may not always be apparent to parents. Parents should be informed of these signs and should report them. Assessment data provide the basis for decision making pertaining to treatment and care concerning infant diarrhea and nutrition. One-to-one teaching that is culturally sensitive and that uses language the caregiver can easily understand is the goal.

Criteria

Home visits are recommended in cases of infants presenting to the emergency room with the following conditions.

1. Acute gastroenteritis (AGE)
2. Vomiting (with no evidence of intestinal obstruction or acute abdomen)
3. Poor intake
4. Dehydration (excluding those patients exhibiting signs of circulatory collapse)

Recommended Visit Pattern

Daily visits are suggested to monitor intake, output, and daily weight; to provide physical assessments; and to ensure compliance with the treatment regime.

PARENT EDUCATION PROGRAM: DIARRHEA

Diarrhea is one of the most common problems in infants, as well as one of the most potentially dangerous. The following information should be helpful in understanding exactly what is going on in the child's body, how to treat diarrhea, and how not to treat diarrhea.

Diarrhea and Dehydration

1. Definition of diarrhea: Three or more liquid stools (liquid bowel movements) in a day.
2. Causes of diarrhea
   a. Germs, bacterial or viral, that cause an infection of the intestines (bowels). This is called gastroenteritis.
   b. Microscopic animal organisms. Giardia is a common cause of a highly contagious diarrhea often transmitted from infant to infant in day care centers.
   c. Fungus (candida is one species) can cause diarrhea, especially in infants who have been weakened by other illnesses or who have immune-deficiency diseases.

   d. Parasitic worms are very common among infants, who tend to put their unwashed fingers and hands in or near their mouths.
   e. Physiologic causes include fever. Many infants get diarrhea along with a cold, change in diet, milk intolerance, or rich or spicy foods.

   Regardless of the cause, diarrhea should stop within a week. If it continues, call the infant's doctor or clinic.

3. Impact of diarrhea on the infant's health
   a. Colds and diarrhea are the two most common illnesses of infants. Worldwide, infants have 1 to 10 episodes of diarrhea a year.
   b. Diarrhea can cause dehydration from fluid loss.
   c. Common diarrhea can cause serious illness or even death, especially in very young infants. In the United States, 200,000 infants per year are hospitalized and 500 infants die as a result of dehydration from diarrhea. This can be prevented if pediatric care providers and caregivers understand diarrhea, dehydration, and simple steps they can take to prevent them.
4. Definition/explanation of dehydration
   a. At birth, the human body is about 80% water. By 9 months, it is 60% water and should stay at that level.
   b. Electrolytes are special kinds of salts (sodium and potassium) in the body that are vital to the body's systems.
   c. Diarrhea causes body fluids and electrolytes to be lost in the stool. This can cause dehydration and even death.
5. Signs of dehydration (indicating a lack of fluid)
   a. Dry mouth (lips or tongue)
   b. Unusual drowsiness, listlessness, or fussiness
   c. Extreme thirst
   d. Sunken-looking eyes
   e. Decreased urination (or less than six wet diapers per day or a period of longer than 4 hours without urination)
   f. Concentrated urine (urine is very dark yellow)
   g. Absence of tears
   h. Rapid heartbeat or pulse
   i. Sunken soft spot (fontanel)
   j. Poor skin turgor (pinch skin on abdomen; the skin should return to normal after being released)
6. What to do if an infant is dehydrated.
   a. If an infant with diarrhea appears dehydrated, has a fever over 101°, cannot drink fluids, or has blood in the stool, call a doctor or clinic ***immediately***. Blood in the stool can make it look red, rust-colored, or flecked with blood.

b. ***If an infant with diarrhea is unconscious, "floppy," or has a high fever (more than 103°), take the infant immediately to the nearest hospital!***

7. Management of gastroenteritis involves three components.
    a. Maintain or restore fluid and electrolyte balance.
    b. Restore the bowel to normal functioning.
    c. Prevent the infection of others in contact with the infant.

8. Care of an infant with diarrhea
   These guidelines will help you to help your infant get well, keep him or her out of the hospital, and avoid a painful needle stick for intravenous treatment.
    a. Rehydration
       To prevent and treat dehydration, start oral rehydration therapy (ORT) as soon as the diarrhea begins. ORT is discussed and explained in detail in the next section.
    b. Feeding
        1) Sometimes people think that it is necessary to "rest the gut" in cases of diarrhea. ***This is not a good practice!*** It is very important that infants eat when they are sick, even when they have diarrhea. Eating the right foods actually helps the infant get well faster. The right foods give the infant the energy needed for healing and for fighting the infection causing the diarrhea. Small, frequent feedings are most often given, yet larger quantities offered less frequently may be recommended because frequent feedings have the potential to induce peristalsis.
        2) ***DO continue to breastfeed or bottlefeed your baby normally*** (unless instructed otherwise by your baby's pediatric care provider).
        3) ***DO NOT give the infant sugary or salty foods or drinks.*** These can make the diarrhea worse.

9. Medication for diarrhea
   Diarrhea is a reaction of the intestines to an infection or irritation. The very best care for most cases of infant diarrhea is simply replacing the fluids and salts lost by giving oral rehydration solution and feeding the infant good foods while he or she is sick or following an illness.

   Parents are usually very concerned about the frequency and appearance of bowel movements and want to give the infant something to "bind" the bowels. This does not really help because, when the infant has diarrhea, the body fluid and salts are still being lost. They are just being held in the intestine longer. The fluid in the intestine does not go back into the body where it is needed! It is possible that the infant is still becoming dehydrated, even though the diarrheal bowel movements are not being expelled. So, "binding" the infant will give parents a false sense of security because it appears that the diarrhea is getting better. It is not—it is just being held inside longer. Also, you might not realize how much fluid is being lost because it is "hidden" in the intestine, so you will not realize how much the infant needs to drink.

   Remember, the main goal is to prevent dehydration and to recognize it early if it does develop.

10. Record keeping
    If your infant has diarrhea it may be helpful to keep a written record, so that if you have to call the pediatric care provider you will be prepared to ask and answer questions. Start the notes as soon as the diarrhea starts. You should record the following information.
    a. Amount and color of the stool and time

b. Amount and kind of fluid the infant takes and time

c. Temperature

d. Weight
If you have a scale, weigh the infant as soon as the diarrhea starts, especially if the infant is under 3 years old. If you have this information when you need to call the doctor, nurse, or clinic, they will be able to decide more easily if the infant should be brought in.

11. Comfort the infant
Infants with diarrhea do not feel well and therefore have special needs. Babies' bottoms hurt and they may be cranky. These are some things you can do to prevent and treat diaper rash to make the baby feel better.

    a. Do not use baby wipes that contain alcohol.

    b. Do change diapers often.

    c. Do wash the infant's bottom with soap, rinse with plain warm water, and gently pat dry.

    d. Do apply Vaseline, Desitin, or A&D ointment to the infant's bottom. This will keep the stool away from the skin.

    e. Do apply cornstarch or baby powder to the infant's bottom.

12. Prevention of diarrhea
The microorganisms (germs) that cause diarrhea are passed by people, objects, and food. To prevent the spread of diarrhea, here are some things you can do.

    a. Wash your hands well with soap and water.

        1) Before cooking food or feeding your infant

        2) After changing your infant's diaper or going to the toilet

        3) After handling raw meat of any kind

        4) After giving a sick infant medication or feeding

    b. Do not let infants play with, or put into their mouths, things that you know are dirty.

    c. Throw disposable diapers out immediately and keep them in a trash can away from infants and pets. The trash can should have a lid.

    d. Keep dirty cloth diapers away from infants and pets and wash them as soon as possible.

    e. Be careful how you store and prepare foods. To prevent the spread of diarrhea from food, be sure to cook and prepare foods correctly and wash dishes and utensils well after use. Foods to be especially careful with are eggs, fish and shellfish, chicken, and pork. Promptly refrigerate foods that can spoil.

Oral Rehydration Therapy (ORT)

1. Definition: Oral rehydration therapy involves drinking a special solution to replace, in the proper proportions, essential body fluids and salts lost during diarrhea to treat and ***prevent dehydration***.

2. Why ORT works: The special salts (electrolytes) and water that are lost in diarrhea are needed by the body to function properly. Drinking a balanced solution of salt, water, and sugar can prevent as well as treat dehydration of people with diarrhea. These solutions are called oral rehydration solutions (ORS) or oral electrolyte solutions (OES).

3. For the solution to work best, proper amounts of the ingredients are critical. Too little or too much of any of the ingredients will cause the solution to not work correctly. (This is why an infant with diarrhea should not have salty or sugary foods and drinks and why plain water is not enough.) However, fluids are critical, and oral rehydration solution is the best replacement fluid. If ORS is not available, then any fluid is better than none.

4. Oral rehydration solutions
   a. What they are
      1) Oral rehydration solutions are special mixtures of water and electrolytes in the correct quantities that will replace the fluids and salts lost in diarrhea.
      2) Commercial brands of ORS are available, including Pedialyte, Ricelyte, and generic brands, which can be found in grocery stores and drug stores.
      3) ***There is also a solution that you can make at home*** that is a good substitute for commercial brands when it is made according to the directions. It is very ***easy*** and ***inexpensive*** to make; the recipe is provided below.
   b. How and when to give them to infants
      1) ***How*** you give the solution is as important as what you give to an infant. To prevent dehydration it is necessary to replace the fluid and salts lost in the stool, so it is important to give enough solution.
      2) When an infant has diarrhea, he or she may have an upset stomach. It is very important to give the solution slowly enough that it can be absorbed by the body and not cause the infant to vomit. Here is a general guide to giving an oral rehydration solution.
         (a) Encourage the infant to take the solution after each stool or every few minutes.
         (b) The solution should be taken in small amounts, either in sips or by spoon, so that it is easily absorbed. Do not let the infant gulp it down.
         (c) An infant under 24 months may need 1/4 to 1/2 cup. A child 2 to 10 years old may need 1/2 to 1 cup.
      3) Remember, the solution is replacing what is lost in the diarrhea, so if there is a lot of diarrhea, be sure to give enough of the oral rehydration solution after each stool.
      4) If the infant vomits, keep giving the solution, but give it in sips of 1/2 to 1 teaspoon every few minutes. This will allow time for it to be absorbed. The rate may need to be slower than before the infant vomited.
      5) When people have the correct amount of fluids and salts in their systems, they urinate often and their urine is clear to light yellow in color. If an infant's urine is dark yellow or the infant is not urinating as much as usual, you may wish to give more oral rehydration solution. Call the doctor or clinic if this condition continues.
   c. How to make homemade cereal-based ORS (the sugar is replaced in this solution by the cereal, which is a complex sugar)

Grandma's ORS Recipe

1/2 to 1 cup of precooked baby rice cereal
2 cups of water
1/4 teaspoon of table salt

Mix all of the ingredients together until well mixed. Be sure to use a level measuring teaspoon. Make the mixture as thick as is drinkable.

Give it a little at a time, give it often, and give as much as the infant will take. (Give a little every minute if the infant will take it.) You can offer Grandma's ORS with a spoon or a cup. Remember, no gulping. Do not give too much; salt can be dangerous. Remember the idea of replacing fluid: one cup out, one cup in. In other words, the amount of diarrhea that comes out is the amount of fluid that should be put back in.

The ORS solution should be covered and stored in the refrigerator if possible. The solution should be discarded after 6 to 8 hours, or when it is too thick to drink.

Reminder: This is not considered food, and the infant should also be encouraged to eat a normal diet of breast milk, formula, and/or recommended foods.

HOME CARE PROTOCOL: ADMINISTRATION OF NEONATAL INTRAVENOUS ANTIBIOTIC

Eligibility Requirements

1. The initial acute treatment has been completed and a decision has been made by pediatric provider to complete therapy course at home.
2. Laboratory values are within the normal range.
3. There are no underlying complications.
4. Parents have demonstrated the ability to cope with home intravenous (IV) therapy.
5. The predischarge assessment in the home has been completed.
6. All of the necessary equipment has been ordered.
7. A feeding pattern has been established.
8. The infant has been discharged within 24 to 48 hours after meeting the discharge criteria.
9. The electric company has been notified of the medical need for power priority.
10. The appropriate utilities have been notified of the need for water, phone, electricity, and heat in cases of economic hardship.
11. An emergency transport plan is in place.

General Nursing and Pediatric Care Provider Treatment Orders

Before discharge of the infant from the hospital, a predischarge evaluation will be completed. This evaluation includes the following areas:

1. Socioeconomic evaluation
2. Laboratory test results
3. Appropriate equipment and supplies ordered and the delivery date scheduled with the parents/caregivers
4. Complete physical assessment to include the following:
    a. Pertinent past and current findings
    b. Appropriate identifying information
        1) Infant's name, address, and phone number
        2) Parents' names
        3) Referring pediatric provider's name, address, and phone number
        4) Insurance types and numbers
        5) Known drug allergies
        6) Type of home care, visits, and frequency

5. Notification of the electric company of the state of medical priority for any child using medical electrical equipment in case of a power outage

6. Notification of the appropriate utilities of the need for water, phone, heat, and electricity in cases of economic hardship

7. Establishment of an emergency transport plan with the family and the appropriate local transport team

Nursing Assessment Each Visit

The nurse will perform a physical assessment and examination to evaluate the areas listed below:

1. Cardiovascular: Assess heart rate, rhythm, and presence of murmur. Palpate peripheral pulses and observe for edema.

2. Respiratory: Auscultate lungs for rate, rhythm, and abnormal breath sounds. Observe the character of respiratory effort (retractions, grunting, or flaring).

3. Metabolic: Assess the infant's temperature and intake (subnormal or above normal).

4. Gastrointestinal: Assess for nausea, vomiting, and diarrhea as signs of antibiotic intolerance. Obtain daily weights. Assess for presence of bowel sounds.

5. Genitourinary: Determine the frequency of voiding. Determine the number of wet diapers per 24 hours.

6. Musculoskeletal: Assess muscle tone, vigor, activity, and movement of all extremities. Change the dressing, if needed.

Intravenous Site

1. Be sure the IV site remains free of signs of infiltration or phlebitis.

2. Restart the IV when infiltration and phlebitis are present.

3. Apply a warm soak for comfort after removing the old IV.

Activity

1. The infant is to be held during feeding, not propped with a bottle.

2. At times other than feeding, provide activity appropriate to the infant's developmental stage.

3. Provide adequate rest periods on a consistent schedule.

Diet

Formula will be determined by the pediatric provider; provide on demand. Be sure to give formula at least every 4 hours.

Education

1. Safety
    a. Review infant/child safety; identify and correct hazards in the home.
    b. Review signs of infection and feeding intolerance.
    c. Stress the importance of follow-up care.
2. Intravenous site care
    a. Avoid bumping or other abuse of the site.
    b. Review the signs of infiltration and phlebitis and the measures to be taken.
    c. Keep the site clean and dry.
3. Growth and development
    a. Review infant development and stimulation to promote growth.
    b. Reinforce the need for immunizations and follow-up visits.
4. Medications: Educate the family concerning the signs and symptoms of adverse reactions to medications prescribed.

Nursing Visit Plan

1. The course of treatment varies from 7 to 21 days, depending upon infection and the discretion of the pediatric care provider.
2. The frequency of administration varies, depending on infant size, age, and the antibiotic used.
3. Nursing visits will be provided as per the pediatric care provider's plan of care. See Box 5-1 for a sample Individual Treatment Plan.

BOX 5-1: INDIVIDUAL TREATMENT PLAN

Infant name: ______________________________

Doctor name: ______________________________

Protocol: Neonatal Administration of Intravenous Antibiotics

Medication order: ______________________________

EQUIPMENT ORDER

1. #22 or #24 intravenous catheters
2. T connectors
3. B& D caps
4. Alcohol swabs
5. Tape
6. Arm boards
7. Heparinized sodium for flush
8. 3 cc syringes
9. 1 cc syringes
10. IV pump
11. IV pole
12. Extension tubing
13. Sterile water for injection
14. Single-use vials of sterile saline for injection (for infants, sterile saline with no preservatives should always be used)
15. Vials of antibiotics
16. 50 cc bags of D5W, or D5NSS for older child
17. 20 cc syringes
18. 250 cc bags of DSW for infant and toddler administration
19. Three-way stop cocks
20. Gloves
21. Needle disposal receptacle

Other equipment: ______________________________

Lab test order: Serum toxicology antibiotic level as ordered.

Diet order: ______________________________

Activity order: ______________________________

HOME CARE PROTOCOL: DRUG WITHDRAWAL/NEONATAL ABSTINENCE SYNDROME (NAS)

Eligibility Requirements

1. The initial acute treatment has been completed.
2. Laboratory test values are within the normal range.
3. The newborn is free of infection.
4. The parents are able to perform the following tasks:
   a. Care for the infant's physical and nutritional needs
   b. Administer medication correctly
5. A social service evaluation has been completed.
6. The infant is taking adequate nutrition for his or her size and averaging a weight gain of 15 to 20 grams per 24 hours over 1 week.
7. A predischarge assessment of the home has been completed.
8. The newborn has been discharged 24 to 48 hours after meeting the discharge criteria.
9. The electric company has been notified of the medical need for power priority.

General Nursing and Pediatric Care Provider Treatment Orders

Before discharge of the newborn from the hospital, a predischarge evaluation will be completed. This evaluation includes the following:

1. Socioeconomic evaluation, with definite reference to the mother's reliability and supports
2. Home health aide needs based upon assessment of the mother's reliability and supports
3. Laboratory test results
4. Neonatal testing results
5. Complete physical assessment and history to include the following areas:
   a. Birth history and hospital course
   b. Appropriate identifying information
      1) Newborn's name, address, phone number
      2) Parents' names
      3) Referring pediatric care provider's name, address, phone number
      4) Insurance type and numbers
      5) Type of home care, visits, and frequency

c. Medications and dietary/treatment orders
d. Supplies and equipment needed
e. Evaluation of initial visit, establishing long-term and short-term goals
f. Signature of the pediatric nurse and date the predischarge assessment was rendered

6. Notification of the electric company of the state of medical priority for any newborn using medical electrical equipment in case of a power outage

7. Notification of the appropriate utilities of the need for water, phone, electricity, and heat in cases of economic hardship

8. Establishment of an emergency transport plan with the family and the appropriate local transport team.

Nursing Assessment Each Visit

The nurse will perform physical assessment and examination to evaluate the following:

1. Cardiovascular: Assess heart rate, rhythm, and presence of murmur. Palpate peripheral pulses and observe for edema. Note the skin color for any molting.

2. Respiratory: Auscultate lungs for rate, rhythm, and abnormal breath sounds. Observe the character of respiratory effort (retractions, grunting, or flaring).

3. Metabolic: Assess the newborn's temperature and intake.

4. Gastrointestinal: Assess for vomiting, frequent loose stools, and irritation of buttocks. Weigh the infant, measure girth, and auscultate bowel sounds. Note that constipation may indicate overuse of paregoric.

5. Genitourinary: Determine the number of wet diapers per 24 hours.

6. Musculoskeletal: Check muscle tone, vigor of activity, and movement of all extremities.

7. Neurologic: Assess the fontanel, irritability, cry, moro reflex, presence of jitters, or seizure activity, inability to quiet, yawning, or sneezing.

Activity

1. Stimulation by excess noise and activity should be minimized.

2. The infant should be kept swaddled in a quiet room with subdued lights.

3. Review measures for minimizing irritability.

Diet

1. Daily quantity will be determined by the pediatric care provider.

2. Document the formula amount and number of feeds per day.

3. Burp frequently to minimize vomiting.

Education

1. Safety
   a. Review infant safety; identify and correct hazards in the home.
   b. Review the signs of infection, feeding intolerance, and seizures with parents.
2. Growth and development
   a. Review infant development and stimulation to promote growth.
   b. Reinforce the need for immunizations and follow-up visits.
3. Drugs: Educate the family concerning the signs and symptoms of adverse reactions to any medication prescribed.
4. Social: Follow up and provide a social service evaluation if there is a drug dependence situation in the family.
5. Miscellaneous: Inform the parents of the community resources available.

HOME CARE PROTOCOL: HOME STAPLE REMOVAL

Nurses may remove staples from women following cesarean section if they have demonstrated to the employing agency that they are technically proficient in staple removal. The following protocol is to be used.

1. Staples will be removed on the fifth postoperative day unless otherwise specified.
2. The client should be afebrile.
3. The wound is to be inspected before staple removal.
4. Do not begin staple removal under the following circumstances:
   a. The client is febrile.
   b. The wound is unusually tender, indurated, or erythematous.
5. If client has a fever or an unusual wound exam, call the OB care provider from the home for a consultation and if you are unable to reach the OB care provider, refer the client to the hospital emergency room.
6. Every other staple is to be removed in sequence.
7. Discontinue staple removal under the following circumstances:
   a. The skin edge opens.
   b. Drainage from the wound appears.
   c. Any staple is unable to be removed.
8. If the skin edge opens or there is drainage from wound, apply a dressing and call the OB care provider from the home for a consultation. If you are unable to reach the OB care provider refer the client to the hospital emergency room.
9. If you are unable to remove staples, refer the client to the OB care provider, to be seen at the office within 72 hours of your visit.
10. Apply steri-strips to the wound at the completion of staple removal.
11. Instruct the client in wound care, signs and symptoms of infection, and removal of steri-strips.

POLICY AND PROCEDURE: THE CLIENT WITH SUDDEN WOUND DEHISCENCE

PURPOSE: Appropriate emergency nursing intervention will be provided in the event of sudden wound dehiscence.

RATIONALE: Appropriateness of action is crucial in preventing further client morbidity.

PREPARATION OF CLIENT:

- Approach the situation calmly, informing the client of all activities. Provide emotional and physical support.
- Assist the client in preparation of needs for hospital transport.

EQUIPMENT:

1. Sterile dressings
2. Sterile normal saline for irrigation
3. Sterile gloves

PROCEDURE:

1. Stay with the client and have someone in the household contact the OB care provider. The nurse should have a family member stay with the client while she is speaking directly to the OB care provider.
2. Have the family notify paramedic, emergency medical technician (EMT), or police transport.
3. If the intestines are exposed, cover with sterile, moist dressings.
4. Keep the client on absolute bed rest until emergency transport arrives.
5. The client may be instructed to bend her knees for relief of tension on the abdomen.
6. Assure the client that the wound will be properly cared for; keep her quiet and relaxed.
7. Instruct the family to gather the appropriate belongings for client hospitalization.
8. The nurse should accompany the client to the hospital if the transport team does not have a nurse, paramedic, or EMT.
9. If the transport team consists of a nurse, paramedic, or EMT, the home care nurse should provide a complete report to this person.
10. The home care nurse will notify his or her supervisor as soon as possible from the client's home.

DOCUMENTATION AND REPORTING:

1. Document all communication and actions taken on the nursing progress notes and the incident report.

2. The nursing supervisor must be notified.

3. The nursing supervisor will follow through with the hospital concerning the client's condition.

4. The nursing supervisor will assure appropriate documentation by the home care nurse.

HOME CARE PROTOCOL: BEREAVEMENT VISIT

Eligibility Requirements

1. Loss of neonate after delivery
2. Previous maladjustment to loss of neonate, infant, or child
3. Referral from social service at client's institution

General Nursing and OB Care Provider Treatment Orders

Before the nursing visit, the nurse will make the following preparations:

1. Consult with the OB care provider and social service.
   a. Obtain the client's physical and psychosocial history.
   b. Assess the availability of family support.
   c. Obtain interpretation of the client's and family's ability to go through the grieving process.
2. Obtain information from the following organizations (whichever are applicable) for support:
   a. National SIDS Foundation
   b. The International Guild for Infant Survival
   c. Society of the Compassionate Friend
   d. The Center of Death Education and Research
   e. Caring Unlimited
   f. Parenting Association
   g. Any other local support group for grieving
3. Obtain important identifying information:
   a. Client's name, address, and phone number
   b. Religion, age, gravida, and parity
   c. Case history
   d. Insurance types and number
   e. Any drug allergies
   f. Schedule for the visit
   g. Name of social worker involved

Nursing Visit

1. Make a socioeconomic evaluation:
   a. Assess whether there is adequate family support.
   b. Assess the grieving process of the family.

2. Identify the grieving process:
    a. Denial and avoidance
    b. Anger
    c. Depression
    d. Rationalization
    e. Acceptance
3. Support the client through the following actions:
    a. Touching
    b. Listening
    c. Reassuring that what they are feeling is OK.
4. Assess for somatic and emotional distress:
    a. Chest pain
    b. Weakness
    c. Sighing
    d. Fainting
5. In dealing with the anger stage (possible accusations against medical technology/hospital/OB care provider/nurse) keep the following points in mind:
    a. Don't be defensive.
    b. Remain calm.
    c. Help the client vent anger.
6. Report to OB care provider after the total evaluation of the grieving visit.
7. A social service consultation may be necessary after the nursing evaluation.

Activity

There are no limitations to activity.

Education

1. Teach the client and family the stages of the grieving period.
2. Support counseling as needed by the client and other family members
3. Provide educational material on grieving.
4. Supply the names and phone numbers of other families who have been in a similar situation for support.

Diet

1. Provide nutritional teaching.
2. Encourage the client to maintain a good, nutritionally balanced diet.

Follow-Up Care

1. Establish with the client that the OB care provider appointment must still be maintained.
2. It may be necessary for social service to follow client.

Medication

1. Medication should be taken only as prescribed by the OB care provider.
2. During the visit review the proper administration of medication, any side effects, and actions of medication.
3. Review the contraindications of any new medication the client may be taking.

POLICY AND PROCEDURE: MEASURES TO LIMIT INCIDENCE OF INFECTIONS IN THE HOME

POLICY: Home care staff members will implement infection control procedures, as necessary.

PURPOSE:
- To control the spread of infection.
- To protect individuals from the transmission of communicable/infectious diseases.

PROCEDURE:

1. Home care staff members will implement infection control procedures with regard to clients, staff, and their environment.
2. Infection control procedures include, but are not limited to, the following measures:
   a. Handwashing by home care staff members in the following situations:
      1) Before and after providing direct client care
      2) After handling soiled or contaminated materials
      3) After using the lavatory
      4) After coughing or sneezing

   b. Following appropriate client wound and skin dressing techniques

   c. Practicing appropriate client skin care

   d. Handling and disposing of client waste products appropriately

   e. Covering nose and mouth when coughing or sneezing

   f. Covering cuts on fingers or hands with clean Band-aids

   g. Taking sick leave days in the following instances:
      1) Any infectious condition
      2) Fever
      3) Diarrhea
      4) Active herpes that is open and weeping (for direct caregivers only)
3. Environmental infection control procedures include, but are not limited to, the following measures:
   a. Maintaining a clean work environment, for example, by maintaining clean counters, tables, and shelves

   b. Keeping clean and dirty items separate

   c. Keeping the client environment clean, neat, and orderly
4. Home care staff members should provide information to all clients regarding infection control principles and procedures, as appropriate.

POLICY AND PROCEDURE: BODY FLUIDS PRECAUTIONS

POLICY: The Centers for Disease Control (CDC) and Occupational Safety and Health Administration (OSHA) recommendations for prevention of exposure to hepatitis B virus (HBV) and human immunodeficiency virus (HIV) will be followed.

PURPOSE:

1. To prevent direct inoculation of infectious material to self or others.
2. To comply with the most recent recommendations for infection control from CDC, which calls for the use of gloves and, if necessary, gowns, masks, and goggles when handling blood or body fluids in the care of all clients.
3. To inform staff of the following OSHA definitions of Standard Precautions and Body Fluids:
   a. Standard Precautions: The term "Standard Precautions" refers to a system for infectious disease control which assumes that every direct contact with body fluids is infectious, and requires every employee exposed to direct contact with body fluids to be protected as though such body fluids were HBV or HIV infected. Therefore, Standard Precautions are intended to prevent health care workers from parenteral mucous membrane and nonintact skin exposures to blood-borne pathogens.
   b. Body Fluids: Fluids that have been recognized by CDC as directly linked to the transmission of HIV or HBV, or to which Standard Precautions apply: blood, semen, blood products, vaginal secretions, cerebrospinal fluid, synovial fluid, pleural fluid, peritoneal fluid, pericardial fluid, amniotic fluid, and concentrated HBV or HIV viruses.

EQUIPMENT:

1. Gloves
2. "Baggies"
3. Labels

The need for gowns, masks, or goggles is determined by the following: if the quantity of body fluids, or the inability to control the loss of body fluids, presents the risk that the face would be sprayed or clothes contaminated.

PROCEDURES: To prevent exposure to body fluids, all nurses must wear gloves at all times when they might come in contact with blood, semen, urine, feces, saliva, lochia, breastmilk, or wounds. Gloves should also be worn when using instruments for vascular access or having direct contact with articles that have been contaminated.

1. Hands should be washed before and after direct contact with the client or secretions.
2. Gowns should be worn when having contact with the client's blood, carrying out procedures in which excessive blood spills or spatters may occur, or using instruments that may became contaminated due to direct contact with blood or secretions (exam instruments).

3. Masks are not necessary for normal client contact including venipuncture. However, use of masks may be necessary if there is a risk of blood being spattered.

4. Articles such as books, magazines, and toys require no special precautions unless visibly contaminated with blood or secretions.

5. Sphygmomanometer and stethoscope require no special precautions unless visibly contaminated.

6. Thermometers should be disinfected with 0.2% iodine or 70% to 90% alcohol, or a thermometer cover should be used.

7. All specimens of body fluids should be put in a well-constructed container with a secure lid to prevent leaking during transport to the lab; the container must then be bagged. If outside contamination of the bag is likely, a second bag must be added.

8. Special precautions should be taken when blood is collected from clients. Disposable needles and syringes must be used. Used needles should not be recapped.

9. Used needles and any discarded blood should be placed in a prominently labeled, impervious, puncture-resistant container designated for this purpose. Do not intentionally break or bend by hand. The medical supply company will pick up the needle box when it is full.

CHAPTER 6

Family Education Materials

The teaching material found in this chapter is meant to to copied and distributed to home care nurses and the families they assist. These are only a few of the teaching tools one can access with a little research. Excellent materials can be found through The Division of Maternal Child Health, Health and Human Services (5600 Fishers Lane, Rockville, MD 20857). In addition, further resources should be available through state and local health departments. Visual and written aids assist the nurse in the education process by stimulating multiple senses and thus increasing stimulation of the memory.

Keep in mind that these items are simply *tools*. They are meant to assist in the educational process. They are not a substitute for the nurse–client relationship that develops out of a nurse's empathy with the client. The nurse should always take the time to review these handouts with clients. Do not assume the client can read or has developed an adequate trusting relationship with you to value your information. Nurses in home care work in the domain of the client, not in the office or the hospital. The client maintains more control in home care because the nurse works on the client's "turf." The nurse's ability to communicate and develop the "helping relationship" is crucial to successful practice of home health nursing.

PARENT EDUCATION PROGRAM: KEGEL EXERCISES

The primary muscle involved in Kegel exercises is the pubococcygeus (P-C) muscle. Exercising the P-C muscle provides the following benefits.

1. Urinary sphincter control is strengthened.
2. Muscle tone in the vagina is increased.
3. The ability to constrict the vagina voluntarily is also increased. This increases female vaginal perception and response during penile–vaginal intercourse.
4. Exercising the P-C muscle contributes to the elimination of pain during sexual intercourse.
5. Exercising the P-C muscle increases the ability to relax the pelvic floor, which aids in the birth of the baby.
6. Kegel exercises also speed up the postpartum recovery of pelvic floor muscle tone.

To identify the P-C muscle, sit on the toilet with your legs spread as far apart as possible. Start and stop the flow of urine. The P-C muscle is the only one that can accomplish this while in this position. Contract the P-C muscle, hold for 3 seconds, relax, and repeat this process. Because the P-C is a muscle like other muscles, with overly strenuous exercise it can become sore. If this happens, either stop doing the exercise for 1 or 2 days until the temporary soreness disappears and then resume, or reduce substantially the number of exercises done per day and then gradually increase to the recommended number.

Once you learn where the P-C muscle is, Kegel exercises can be done during daily activities that do not involve a great deal of moving around (e.g., driving an automobile, sitting, doing dishes, watching TV, waiting in a checkout line, lying in bed). Practice the Kegel exercises five times a day (15 contractions each time) or 10 contractions each time you open the refrigerator. Soon Kegels will become second nature to you.

PARENT EDUCATION PROGRAM: POSTPARTUM INSTRUCTIONS FOR MOTHERS

Rest

1. The new mother should get plenty of rest for the first couple of weeks.
2. The client should care for herself and her baby only; she shouldn't expect too much of herself.
3. The new mother should obtain help for general household duties (cleaning, cooking, laundry, shopping, and caring for older children).
4. Emphasize that the new mother needs to rest when the baby is sleeping.
5. Limit visitors to relatives and close friends.
6. Remember, fatigue decreases the milk supply and the ability to cope with new and added responsibilities.

Activity

1. Limit stair climbing for the first week.
2. The client should let her body be the guide for activity and exercise.
3. The new mother may go out to dinner or for a ride but she should not drive for 1 to 2 weeks unless otherwise instructed by her physician. Cesarean section patients should verify with their OB care provider when driving is permitted.

Diet

1. Advise the client to drink 8 to 10 glasses of water per day.
2. Her diet should consist of protein, fruits, vegetables, and milk.
3. A small bowl of bran daily will prevent constipation
4. The client should continue taking prenatal vitamins daily at least until the postpartum exam. If the OB care provider has not instructed her to do so, the client should verify this with her physician.
5. An adequate diet as shown above is important, particularly if the mother is breastfeeding, because it takes about 800 calories daily to produce the milk the baby needs.
6. Remember, if the new mother does not eat, she will become fatigued and milk volume will decrease.

Vaginal Discharge

1. At first discharge is red, like a heavy period, for 1 to 3 days.
2. By the 3rd day the discharge should have thinned and lightened in color.
3. By the 10th day the discharge is often a pale pink, watery fluid, heavy enough to wear a light pad.
4. If, after the 3rd day, bleeding becomes bright red and heavy again, it is often a sign that the new mother has done too much and should slow down and rest.

Intercourse

1. For the majority of women, intercourse may be resumed when the vaginal area feels comfortable and the episiotomy has healed. She should check any doubts with her physician.
2. Gentleness and added lubrication may be needed for comfort when sexual activity is first resumed.
3. Breastfeeding mothers may ovulate before their first menstrual period, therefore it is possible to get pregnant again even before menstruation has resumed.
4. Foam and condoms will provide contraception if sexual activity is resumed before 6 weeks postpartum.
5. Birth control can be discussed at the 6-week postpartum visit.

Baths and Showers

1. The new mother may shower as necessary, but stress two points. ***Do not*** take a tub bath for at least 3 days unless otherwise instructed by the OB care provider. ***Do not*** use bubble bath or oils in the bath water.
2. Warm showers may help to relieve the discomfort of breast engorgement.
3. ***Do not use douches!!!***

Stitches and Hemorrhoids

1. Warm tub baths or sitz baths are recommended several times a day.
2. For discomfort of hemorrhoids use Nupercainol cream, Dermoplast, or Tucks pads. The client should consult her OB care provider.
3. There is no cause for alarm if a week or two postpartum loose stitches are found on a pad or in the toilet.
4. Reassure the new mother that stitches normally are absorbed or loosen when they no longer are needed.

Postpartum Blues

1. The new mother may experience postpartum blues during the first 10 days postpartum. The most common symptom is unexpected and unexplainable crying. Also, she may feel irritable.
2. Postpartum blues usually go away about 72 hours after onset, but they may continue for as long as 10 days.
3. If postpartum blues symptoms persist or increase in severity, they may be an early sign of postpartum depression.
4. Postpartum depression is experienced by 10% of all women and may occur anywhere within 6 months after delivery.
5. Signs and symptoms of postpartum depression
   a. Sleep disturbances may occur.
   b. Loss of appetite is common.
   c. Fear and anxiety are also signs of postpartum depression.
   d. A feeling of hopelessness may develop.
   e. Hostility or self-blame are also common.
   f. Difficulty concentrating or making decisions is another sign.
6. The client may want to seek professional help if the signs and symptoms of postpartum depression are experienced.

Baby's Fussy Periods

1. The baby may go through fussy periods during the day or evening.
2. Fussy periods may happen because the mother's milk supply is low at the end of the day.
3. The new mother may need to nurse more frequently.
4. Use calming tactics such as rocking, walking, strollers, swings, etc.
5. Lay the baby down to see if he or she will sleep.

Postpartum Problems

Call your health care provider if any of the following problems occur.

1. A flulike feeling, fever, or chills
2. A foul-smelling discharge or unusual abdominal tenderness
3. Redness and tenderness of the breasts
4. Extreme tenderness of the episiotomy area

5. Tenderness of the pubic bone, accompanied by frequency, urgency, and burning with urination

These symptoms may indicate an infection of some type, which requires professional attention and treatment.

PARENT EDUCATION PROGRAM: NEWBORN INSTRUCTIONS

Bathing

1. Sponge bathe the newborn with mild soap (low alkaline) such as Dove or Castille until the cord has fallen off and the area is completely healed.
2. Do not use oil or powder on the baby's head or skin.
3. When the navel is healed, the baby may have a tub bath.
4. Bathe the baby before feeding.

Cord Care

1. The cord usually falls off within 7 to 10 days.
2. Use alcohol and cotton to cleanse and bathe the area around the base of the cord at every diaper change.
3. There may be one or two drops of blood when the cord separates.
4. Keep the diaper folded beneath the navel to facilitate drying of the cord.
5. Call the pediatric care provider if the cord has a foul odor or if the skin of the abdominal area around the umbilical cord becomes red.

Diaper Rash

1. Change the baby's diaper when it is soiled.
2. Avoid using plastic pants when possible or change the baby frequently. Air the buttocks when changing.
3. Diapers should be washed with mild soap and rinsed well after each laundering.
4. Apply Balmex or Desitin to the diaper area, especially the creases, at each diaper change (Vaseline can be used all the time on the diaper area).

Circumcision

Apply Vaseline liberally at every diaper change until the area is no longer red or swollen.

Nails

1. Use an emery board to file nails. They are too soft to cut with scissors for the first couple of weeks.
2. Never cut with cuticle scissors

Clothing

1. Keep the baby warm, but do not overheat.
2. Use simple, easily washed clothes.
3. On hot days, a diaper and T-shirt may be enough.
4. The baby should wear one more layer of clothing than his or her mother.
5. If it is cool and breezy, the baby's head should be covered.

Feeding

1. If breastfeeding, refer to instructions and information on breastfeeding.
2. Hold the baby at every feeding.
3. Feed the baby when he or she is hungry (usually every 3 to 5 hours).
4. Do not wake the baby at night.
5. Burp the baby after every $^1/_2$ to 1 ounce at first.
6. Place the baby on his or her stomach or right side (roll the blanket and place behind the back for support).

   "Recent research shows that SIDS is more common in babies who go to sleep on their tummies. By making sure your baby goes to sleep on its back or side, you can help reduce the risk of SIDS" (*Back to Sleep: Reducing the Risk of Sudden Infant Death Syndrome—What You Can Do.* U.S. Public Health Service, the American Academy of Pediatrics, the SIDS Alliance, and the Association of SIDS Program Professionals). If you have any questions about your baby's sleep position, contact your health care provider first. Then you can call, toll free, 1-800-505-CRIB, or write to Back to Sleep, P.O. Box 29111, Washington DC 20040, for more information.

7. Do not start any new foods (cereal, juice, or fruit) until the pediatric care provider gives permission.
8. Use formula as ordered by the pediatric care provider. The powdered form may be more economical. The client should always follow the instructions on the can for mixing and preparing the formula.
9. The baby may have 1 to 2 ounces of boiled, cooled water if fussy.

Bowel Movements

1. The breastfed baby's bowel movements are normally loose and unformed.
2. The breastfed baby may have several small movements each day or may go for several days without having a bowel movement at all.
3. A totally breastfed baby is never constipated and seldom has diarrhea (watery bowel movements). Relax with your infant. He or she will adjust to you. If you are tense, the baby will feel tense; if you are relaxed, it will help relax your baby.

PARENT EDUCATION PROGRAM: BREASTFEEDING

Position for Breastfeeding

1. Assume a comfortable position (sitting, lying, football hold); positions should be rotated to avoid stress or sore nipples.
2. Bring the baby to the nipple. You may want to use pillows. This avoids the stress of the baby pulling on the nipples.
3. Expose the breast. Support the baby's head in the crook of the arm, with the other hand supporting the nipple in a scissorslike hold or thumb and forefinger hold.
4. Compress the breast if it is large, with the finger at the baby's nose to prevent obstruction of breathing.
5. Timing
   a. Feed for 5 minutes per side on the first day.
   b. Feed for 7 to 8 minutes per side on the second day.
   c. Feed for 10 minutes per side on the third day.
   d. Build up to 20 minutes per side.
   e. If the baby falls asleep at 10 minutes, when milk comes in cut back to 5 minutes per side.
   f. If the baby is still hungry, you may go back to the first side for another 5 minutes.
   g. Nurse both breasts at each feeding. Start with the breast you ended with at the last feeding.
   h. At end of the feeding, break the suction by placing your finger in the corner of the baby's mouth.
   i. Air dry the nipples after each feeding and apply Eucerin cream around the areola (brown area) but not on the tip of the nipple. This will keep the nipples from becoming tender.

Breast Massage and Hand Expression

1. Breast massage must be used to bring the milk down to the baby, to relieve fullness, and before pumping or hand expressing to decrease the time spent on collection. (See Table 6-1.)

TABLE 6-1.
Breast Pumping Schedule

	Right Breast	Left Breast	Right Breast	Left Breast
Day 1	2 min	2 min	2 min	2 min
Day 2	3 min	3 min	3 min	3 min
Day 3	4 min	4 min	4 min	4 min
Day 4	5 min	5 min	5 min	5 min

2. To massage: Place one hand under the breast. With the other hand, stroke down toward the nipple, starting from the shoulder. Then stroke under the breast and up. Do this for 1 minute.

3. To hand express: Put the thumb and forefinger on the areola about 1 inch from the nipple. Press back toward the chest wall and squeeze together to compress the milk sinus.

Milk Collection and Storage

1. Milk may be collected and stored when mothers work or are not going to be home for feedings and want the baby to drink from a bottle.

2. Collect milk by hand expression, breast pump, or with milk cups. One ounce at a time may be accumulated, so make sure that enough time is allotted.

3. Collect in a clean container.

4. Chill milk, then freeze. Chilled milk may be poured on top of frozen.

5. Milk may be stored in the refrigerator for 24 to 48 hours only.

6. Glass or plastic bottles or double bagged nursers may be used.

7. Milk can be kept in the back of the freezer for several months.

8. To defrost, run under cold, then warm water, then shake.

9. Discard defrosted milk that the baby does not use.

10. Milk to be transported should be placed in an insulated bag, frozen, or packed with ice.

Breastfeeding Solutions and Problems

1. Soreness
   a. Nipples may become red and cracked or bleeding. The nipple may be sore until it becomes accustomed to baby's sucking, or soreness may be due to poor positioning, removing the baby from the breast improperly, not allowing the nipples to dry, or irritants such as soap, shampoo, rough clothing, plastic liners in bras, or harsh laundry detergents.
   b. Solutions
      1) Rotate the position of the baby when feeding.
      2) Provide short, frequent feedings.
      3) Make sure the baby has the large portion of the nipple in the mouth, not just the tip.
      4) Make sure the baby's mouth is close to the nipple to avoid pulling on the nipple.
      5) Air dry the nipples and use Eucerin cream as necessary.
      6) Nurse on the least sore side first.
      7) Always break suction before removing the baby.

8) Try saline soaks, ice on the nipples before feeding, a nipple shield or Vitamin E oil if the nipple becomes cracked or bleeds.

2. Fullness or engorgement
   a. Breasts become full on the second or third day postpartum, when the milk comes in. Engorgement is when the milk becomes backed up and the breast and nipples become hard and shiny.
   b. Solutions
      1) Short, frequent feedings help. Do not miss feedings, and nurse on both sides each feeding.
      2) Warm showers, compresses, massage, and expression relieve the fullness.
      3) Make sure the bra is not cutting or binding in any place.
      4) Occasionally expressing or pumping after feeding may relieve fullness.
3. Plugged duct
   a. A plugged duct produces a lump or tenderness in one spot.
   b. Solution
      1) Nurse on the affected breast first.
      2) Direct the baby's chin toward the lump when nursing.
      3) Avoid tight bras, underwire bras, and bunching clothing.
      4) Use massage and heat while nursing to encourage lump drain.
4. Breast infection
   a. Symptoms: flulike feeling, redness, tenderness and fever. The condition may be aggravated by not emptying the breast completely, abrupt weaning, or the mother's fatigue.
   b. Solutions
      1) Heat: warm, moist compresses may help.
      2) Rest will alleviate the mother's fatigue, helping her condition.
      3) Empty the breast completely; when nursing, direct the baby's chin toward a sore spot or lump.
      4) If the client's temperature increases to 100°, call the physician.

Growth Spurts

1. Growth spurts usually come within the first 10 days, at 3 weeks, at 3 months, and at 6 months.
2. The baby may want to nurse more often.
3. Nurse the baby on demand to build up the milk supply.
4. Do not give supplemental feeding, because this may interfere with establishment of an adequate milk supply. The more frequently the breasts are emptied, the more milk is produced.

PARENT EDUCATION PROGRAM: EXPRESSING BREAST MILK

Breast milk may be expressed and collected for later use by hand expression, a hand-operated breast pump, or a semi-automatic battery-operated or electric breast pump. A sterile container, such as sterile plastic bottle bags (Playtex or Gerber liners) or a sterilized plastic or glass bottle, should be used to collect the milk. Before collecting milk, wash your hands with soap and water and dry them thoroughly.

Massage each breast in this way. If large-breasted, support the breast with one hand. Beginning at the chest wall, use the other flattened hand to exert gentle pressure on the breast toward the nipple, working around the breast. Work in the areas of greatest milk duct development, under the breast and along the side under the arm. Use the palms of the hands, not the fingers, for firm pressure.

Stimulate the let-down reflex or milk ejection reflex by gently rolling and tugging the nipples between your thumb and forefinger. Dripping of milk from the nipples is one sign that the let-down or milk ejection reflex is working. When you feel that the let-down reflex has begun to work, you can begin expressing breast milk by the chosen method.

Collecting milk may take about 20 minutes. Alternate the breast from which you are expressing milk about four times; when the milk flow slows down on one breast, switch to the other breast.

A breast pump collection kit should be washed daily in soap and water and rinsed between uses. A dishwasher (which leaves no soap residue) provides an excellent method for cleaning the kit. When collecting milk for a hospitalized infant, the collection kit must the sterilized daily.

PARENT EDUCATION PROGRAM: STORAGE OF HUMAN MILK

Containers

For hospitalized infants, ask your baby's nurse for storage containers. For home use, the following containers and methods are recommended.

1. Clean heavy plastic or glass containers.
2. Disposable bottle liners; double bags are more sturdy.
3. Seal with a lid or twist tie and store upright until frozen.
4. Label the container with the date on which the milk was expressed

Storage

For hospitalized infants, milk should be refrigerated within 1 hour of expressing. In general, use the following guidelines.

1. Milk may be kept at room temperature.
   a. Colostrum: 12 to 24 hours
   b. Mature milk: 6 to 10 hours

2. Milk may be refrigerated.
   a. Home use: up to 5 days
   b. Hospitalized infants: up to 48 hours
3. Milk may be frozen.
   a. Home use: 2 weeks in a freezer compartment located inside a refrigerator
   b. Home use: 6 months in a refrigerator/freezer with separate doors (frost free)
   c. Home use: 6 months to 1 year in a deep freeze, 0°F or below
   d. Hospitalized infants: 3 months

Warming Milk

Thaw and/or heat milk by placing the container in warm water. Human milk heats to a comfortable feeding temperature in about 10 minutes.

PARENT EDUCATION PROGRAM: HOME PHOTOTHERAPY

1. The unit should be used continuously except when bathing your infant, unless otherwise instructed.
2. A visiting nurse will obtain daily bilirubin blood samples, deliver the samples to a lab, and notify both you and your infant's health care provider of the results.
3. Take your baby's temperature every 8 hours throughout the course of home phototherapy. Because the fiberoptic blanket is not a heat source, temperature instability may signal a problem such as an infection.
4. Monitor the number of wet diapers and record on the flowsheet.
5. Monitor the number and the consistency of bowel movements and record this information on the flowsheet. Your infant may have loose, green-tinged bowel movements as the bilirubin begins to break down.
6. For the bottlefed infant, note and record the amount of formula taken and the frequency of feeding. Feedings should be every 3 hours.
7. For the breastfed infant, note and record the length and frequency of nursing. Feedings should be every 3 hours.
8. Supplement formula or breastfeeding with glucose water unless otherwise instructed.
9. Leave the child on his or her stomach for 1 to 2 hours after eating. Never position the infant on his or her back.
10. The illuminator box should be placed only on a hard, flat surface no more than 4 feet from where the baby will be positioned. Be sure that the air vent in the rear of the unit is not blocked. Use a table or stand next to the baby's bed or the seat where you will be sitting to hold or nurse the baby. Do not put the illuminator next to or on a radiator or heater.
11. Insert the metal collar of the fiberoptic panel completely into the insert of the illuminator. The end of the metal collar of the fiberoptic panel is designed to be even with the end of the insert of the illuminator. Turn the metal collar of the panel clockwise one quarter-turn, to lock it in place.
12. Plug the illuminator box into an electrical outlet. You will need a three-pronged plug (grounded) outlet close by for the electrical cord. A heavy-duty extension cord, such as those used for power tools or appliances, can be used.
13. Insert the panel into a disposable panel cover, ensuring that the light faces the fabric side of the cover, ***not*** the plastic side.
14. Proper placement of the fiberoptic panel will prevent possible skin irritation under the baby's arms. Follow the directions below to assure proper placement:
    a. Place the covered panel around the baby, under his or her arms. Be sure that the fabric side goes against the skin. The lower part of the panel will be on the outside of the baby's diaper. Be sure the diaper is folded down below the baby's navel in front and as far as possible in back so that as much of the skin as possible is exposed to the light.

b. Using two of the tape tabs provided, fasten the panel in place by affixing the tabs on the plastic side of the cover at the open end, close to where you inserted the fiberoptic panel. ***Do not wrap the baby too tightly.*** A good rule of thumb is to place two fingers between the panel and the baby's skin.

c. You can now place a T-shirt on the baby, and wrap the child in a blanket or a sleeper.

d. In larger or more active babies, to prevent possible skin irritation under the baby's arms, tuck a little of the baby's T-shirt, blanket, or sleeper into the top of the panel. Doing this will help cushion the armpit area, preventing skin irritation. You may also use breast shields under the baby's arms.

15. You may now switch on the illuminator and start treatment.

16. You may pick up your baby at any time to hold the child. You can rock, cuddle, or feed the baby. Do not walk around with the baby wrapped in the blanket unit, as you could trip and fall, injuring yourself or the baby. Stay close enough to the illuminator box that it is not pulled off its stand or table.

17. Call your pediatric care provider in the following situations (Box 6-2 is a sample parent information sheet for use in emergencies):

    a. If your child is refusing feedings

    b. If there are persistent temperature control problems

    c. If your child has fewer than five wet diapers over a 24-hour period

    d. If there is a pronounced change in your child's level of activity

    e. If your child vomits entire feedings

BOX 6-2: PARENT INFORMATION SHEET

Pediatric Provider Phone Number: ______________________________

Agency Phone Number: ______________________________

TROUBLESHOOTING: If the fiberoptic panel does not light, check all connections. If it still does not light, call the agency office.

PARENT EDUCATION PROGRAM: INFANT STIMULATION

Infant stimulation is a program of techniques and tools designed to encourage the growth and development of neonates and infants. Infant stimulation is provided to compensate for the limited opportunities that long-term hospitalized infants have or to augment the activities of an average infant. It is a technique that should be based on the four R's of infant stimulation.

1. Rhythm
   All stimulation techniques should be rhythmical, steady, and unforced.

2. Reciprocity
   All infant stimulation should be reciprocal—should involve interaction, "give and take," between the child and the stimulator. The stimulator must be involved.

3. Repetition
   All infant stimulation activities and techniques should involve repetition to promote better learning, to improve neural pathway development, to provide security, and to maintain goals and skills achieved.

4. Reinforcement
   All infant stimulation activities should provide positive and genuine reinforcement of the worth of the infant as an individual. Reinforcement heightens self-esteem and strengthens the bond and attachment between the infant and the stimulator. The infant and stimulator must approach this as fun time.

Infant stimulation has a profound effect upon the mental, physical, and emotional development of each infant. It enhances the mental development of the infant by stimulating curiosity, cultivating a longer attention span, and promoting more age-appropriate play skills. Infant stimulation affects the physical growth of the infant by promoting better muscle coordination and better muscle control, and infants tend to gain weight faster. Emotionally, infants tend to establish strong attachments, trust that their needs will be met, have a sense of control over their environment, smile sooner and more frequently, are content, and have a secure self-image.

Parents should be encouraged to perform infant stimulation activities. Infant stimulation provided in the home by a consistent caretaker is important to the recently hospitalized infant because these infants receive less individual handling and therefore less stimulation. They are separated from their parents for longer time frames, which interferes with the bonding process and lessens the quality of parent–child interaction. They are often deprived of normal newborn experiences.

The infant stimulation program should be based upon the child's present level of functioning and upon the child's needs along the developmental continuum. Often, a child will be functioning well in the areas of cognition, language, or social/emotional development, yet due to confinement the child's motor skills will be delayed. Therefore, each child's program should be tailored to meet his or her individual needs; it should be based upon the child's developmental age and should provide for activity development in each skill area. Activities selected should encourage age-appropriate play skills while taking into consideration the child's medical situation, developmental age, and capabilities. Infants suspected of delays in any of these areas should be referred to the local early intervention program for evaluation.

Below is a list of suggested play activities and toys for the infant, according to age.

1. 1 month: Provide mobiles, rattles, black-and-white objects, and bright simple pictures lining the crib. The baby enjoys leg/arm cycling and smiles at faces.

2. 2 months: The baby enjoys listening to a variety of sounds, therefore talk and sing to him or her often. Lay the baby on his or her stomach and lay on your stomach with your head facing the baby's. Try to get the baby to hold up his or her head and make eye contact. The baby will also respond to voices.

3. 3 months: Peek-a-boo games encourage discovery. Provide soft, safe, furry cuddle toys. Mount a mirror for the baby.

4. 4 months: Allow some time for the baby to play alone. Encourage movement and rolling. The baby will also react to sounds.

5. 5 months: Provide durable, washable toys with handles. Begin "Pat-a-cake" songs and "So Big" games with gestures. Encourage rocking, wriggling, and rolling by placing objects at arm's length away; this will also encourage the baby to reach out and grab.

6. 6 months: Play "Where's baby?" Play knee games and tummy tickles. The baby will like to laugh and squeal.

7. 7 months: Play hold the baby's hands and encourage standing/walking motion.

8. 8 months: Imitate the baby. Chase the baby. Provide pull toys, stacking blocks, and building blocks.

9. 9 months: The baby will enjoy toys to be picked up with the fingers, push/pull toys, and musical toys.

10. 10 months: Baby books, baby blocks, and children's music are appropriate.

11. 11 months: Riding toys pushed by feet and pop-up toys are suitable.

12. 12 months: Push/pull toys, baby books, children's music, and short videos are appropriate.

PARENT EDUCATION PROGRAM: EMERGENCY CARE GUIDE

Important Numbers

Emergency Medical Services: ________________________________

Poison Control Center: ________________________________

Family Doctor: ________________________________

Bites and Stings

Call 911 (or the local emergency number) immediately if a bite wound is bleeding severely. Proceed as for *Bleeding,* described below. Also do this if the wound is deep or from an unknown animal. If the wound is not bleeding profusely, wash the area with mild soap and running water while you wait for help to arrive, but do not use ointments or creams. If any tissue has been bitten off, wrap it in a clean, wet cloth, place it in a plastic bag, and bring it with you to the hospital. If the child has been stung, call 911 (or the local emergency number) if he or she shows signs of a severe allergic reaction such as shock, wheezing, or spreading rash or welts. This can be life-threatening!!!

Bleeding

Try to control the bleeding by applying direct pressure to the wound or cut with a clean cloth. Elevate the wounded area unless you suspect a broken bone. Call 911 (or the local emergency number) if the bleeding cannot be controlled or if there is a puncture wound caused by a large or embedded object. If the wound seems deep or gaping and you suspect the child needs stitches, go to the hospital emergency room.

Broken Bones and Head/Spine Injuries

In situations such as car accidents, falls greater than the child's height, or significant trauma to the head or spine, assume there is a head or spine injury. Call 911 (or the local emergency number) immediately. Do not move the child; keep him or her still. Control any bleeding (see *Bleeding,* above). For broken bones, immobilize the injured part with a splint—only if you have been properly trained in the technique—and call 911 (or the local emergency number).

Burns

1. If burns are on the child's face, hands, feet, or genitals, or if they are white, blistered, or charred, or larger than the size of the child's hand, call 911 (or the local emergency number). While waiting for paramedics to arrive, cover the burns with a clean, cool, wet towel or sheet, or flush with cool water. For open wounds, use a dry towel.

2. For chemical burns, flush the area with running water until help arrives. Remove any of the child's clothing or jewelry saturated with the chemical as soon as possible.

3. For electrical burns or shock, do not touch the child until you have separated him or her from the power source by turning off the electricity. Check breathing and pulse, then call 911 (or the local emergency number).

4. For minor burns, flush the area with cool water and call the family doctor for follow-up care. Never use ointments, creams, or butter without consulting a physician.

Dental Emergencies

Carefully remove any tooth fragments from the mouth. Do not clean the tooth or remove any tissue attached to it; submerge it in a glass of milk (or water if milk is not available) and take both the child and the tooth to the dentist immediately.

Drowning

Begin cardiopulmonary resuscitation as needed on an unconscious child. If the child's pulse has stopped, have someone call 911 (or the local emergency number) while you begin CPR (see *No Pulse* below).

Poisoning

If the child has any extreme symptoms—such as unconsciousness, breathing difficulties, or seizures—call 911 (or the local emergency number). Otherwise, call the area Poison Control Center, specifying the substance involved, how much was ingested, and the child's age, weight, and condition. Have syrup of ipecac on hand, but do not induce vomiting unless instructed to do so. If you are told to go to a hospital, take the poisonous substance container along.

Any First-Aid Situation (except spine injuries)

After you have given specific care, lay the child on his or her back, elevate the legs slightly, and keep his or her body at a comfortable temperature until help arrives.

Choking

1. Infants up to 12 months
    a. If the baby is coughing forcefully, do not interfere or you may make the situation worse; allow the obstruction to clear itself.
    b. If the infant cannot cough, breathe, or cry:
        1) Stand or sit with him face down along your forearm, resting your arm on your thigh so that the baby's head is lower than his chest; cup his jaw with your hand. With the heel of your other hand, give four quick, firm blows to his back between the shoulder blades.
        2) If this does not dislodge the item, turn the baby onto his back, keeping his head lowered. Give four chest thrusts, with two fingers placed on the breastbone one finger's-width below the imaginary line connecting the nipples. Compress the breastbone $1/2$ to 1 inch with each thrust.

3) Repeat the combination of back blows and chest thrusts until the object comes out or until the infant becomes unconscious In either case, have the baby checked later for internal injuries.

c. If the infant loses consciousness, roll the infant onto his or her back; avoid twisting the body and neck. Open the airway by tilting the head back gently. Push down on the forehead until the chin points up and the mouth drops open.

2. Children 12 months and older

   a. If the child is coughing forcefully, talking, or breathing, don't do anything; allow the obstruction to clear itself.

   b. For a conscious child who cannot breathe at all, perform the Heimlich maneuver. Bring your arms around the child from behind. Make a fist, and place the thumb side against the middle of the abdomen just above the navel. Grab your fist with your other hand and press in with quick, upward thrusts. Repeat until the object comes out or the child becomes unconscious.

   c. If the child loses consciousness:

      1) Roll the child onto his or her back; avoid twisting the neck and back. Open the airway by tilting the head back gently. Push down on the forehead while lifting the chin. Look, listen, and feel breathing for 3 to 5 seconds. If the child shows no sign of breathing, pinch the nose shut and cover the mouth with yours. Blow in two puffs of air, taking a breath in between. Watch the chest as you do this; if it does not rise, re-tilt the head and do it again.

      2) If the chest still does not rise, administer blows and thrusts as for *Choking*, above. Then do a foreign-object check. Open the mouth, holding the tongue down with your thumb. If you can see an object (and only if you can see one), remove it by sweeping your little finger with a hook action along the base of the tongue. Repeat the cycle of head-tilt/chin-lift, two breaths, blows and thrusts, and object check until breaths go in.

      3) If breaths do go in, check for a pulse for 5 to 10 seconds with two fingers placed on the inside of the child's upper arm midway between the elbow and the armpit. If there is a pulse, but still no breathing, continue breathing into the mouth and nose once every 3 seconds. If you cannot detect a pulse within 10 seconds, start CPR (see *No Pulse*, below).

No Pulse

1. If the infant is not breathing and has no pulse, give CPR. Place two fingers on the breastbone, one finger's-width below the nipple line. Push the chest downward $1^1/_2$ to 1 inch and release, five times in quick succession (within 3 seconds). Then give one breath (as in *Choking*, item 2.c.1, above). Continue CPR for 1 minute, then recheck the pulse. If there is no pulse, give one rescue breath and continue CPR until the pulse resumes or help arrives.

2. When breaths do go in, check for a pulse on the side of the neck. If there is a pulse but still no breathing, continue breathing into the mouth once every 4 seconds. If you cannot detect a pulse within 10 seconds, start CPR.

Unconsciousness and Choking

Give 6 to 10 quick upward thrusts with the heel of your hand placed just above the navel. Then open the mouth, holding the tongue down with your thumb; if you can see a foreign object, remove it by sweeping your little finger with a hook action along the base of the tongue. Repeat the cycle of head-tilt/chin-lift, two breaths, blows and thrusts, and object check until breaths go in (as in *Choking*, item 2.c.1, above).

PARENT EDUCATION PROGRAM: BASIC HOME SAFETY

Fire Safety (to eliminate fire hazards)

1. The furnace and water heater should be checked at least once a year to ensure safety.
2. Wood stoves or portable heaters should be installed properly, and chimneys should be cleaned and inspected once a year.
3. Flammable liquids should be stored outside, away from any heat source, and disposed of properly.
4. Electrical appliances should be used safely and checked periodically.
5. Matches, cigarettes, and smoking materials should be disposed of safely in an ashtray or fire-resistant container.
6. The kitchen stove should be kept free of grease. No loose-fitting clothes should be worn when cooking. Pot handles should be turned away from the front of the stove and potholders always should be used.
7. Oxygen should be used away from open flames and heat. Do not place concentrator near a heat source. Tubing should not come in contact with stoves, space heaters, or baseboard heating coils. Do not use electrical devices, such as electric razors, while using oxygen. Post "NO SMOKING" signs. Clean up any oil or grease before using oxygen (as it may combine with oxygen and spontaneously ignite).
8. Develop a fire safety plan.
   a. Standard fire regulations recommend one smoke detector on every level of the home.
   b. Develop an evacuation plan for use in case of fire. Note which family members will require assistance because of age, illness, or disability.
   c. Establish clear pathways to all exits. Do not block exits with furniture or boxes.
   d. Have keys stored near doors locked with deadbolts.
   e. Do not leave cooking unattended for long periods of time.
   f. Chimneys should be inspected annually to avoid dangerous buildup of creosote.
   g. Kerosene heaters, wood stoves, and fireplaces should not be left unattended while in use. Never use a gas stove for space heating.
   h. Have a fire extinguisher in an easily accessible place (e.g., kitchen).

Electrical Safety

1. Cords must not be placed beneath furniture or rugs.
2. Replace frayed cords.
3. Do not overload extension cords. Check rating labels on cords and appliances.

4. Multiple outlet adapters should not be used on electrical outlets.
5. Cover unused outlets, and teach young children not to touch plugs, cords, or outlets.
6. Never replace a fuse with a penny or a higher amp fuse. Use correctly sized fuses at all times.
7. Never turn on an appliance or plug one in while standing in water or if your hands are wet.
8. Call a professional electrician if you suspect an electrical problem. Blown fuses or dimmed lights may indicate a wiring problem.
9. Make sure the electrical system is sufficient when using medical equipment such as ventilators and oxygen concentrators. Check with the medical supplier or an electrician.
10. Use three-pronged adapters when required.
11. When ambulating with a pump, IV pole, electrical cord, or IV tubing, carefully position the equipment between you and the outlet, to avoid falls or electrical accidents.

Environmental Safety

1. Loose rugs, runners, and mats should be secured to the floor with double-sided tape or rubber matting.
2. Carpet edges should be tacked down.
3. Torn, worn, frayed carpeting should be repaired, replaced, or removed.
4. Cupboards should be organized so that frequently used items are on lower shelves.
5. A sturdy stepstool should be used to reach items on high shelves.
6. Heavy items should be stored flat on lower levels of the closet to avoid falls and injury.
7. Stairs, hallways, and passageways between rooms should be well lit and free of clutter.
8. Stairs should have sturdy, well-secured handrails on both sides. Install gates, if needed, to protect children from falls.
9. Avoid using stairs while wearing only socks or smooth-soled shoes.
10. Furniture should be arranged to allow free movement in heavy traffic areas.
11. Hazardous tools and firearms should be kept locked up. Unplug appliances and tools when not in use.
12. Cleaning fluids, polishes, bleaches, detergents, and all poisons should be stored separately and clearly marked. Proper ventilation should be available when cleaning fluids are being used.
13. Spills should be cleaned up promptly.
14. Old newspapers and cleaning cloths should not be stockpiled.

15. Insects, rodents, and bad odors should be controlled.

16. Place at least one phone in a position that is accessible in the event that an accident renders a person unable to stand. Emergency numbers should be posted near the phone, including ambulance, doctor, fire, police, and poison control.

17. Entrance ways should be clear of leaves, snow, and ice.

Bathroom Safety

1. Tubs and showers should have a textured surface or nonskid mats or strips to prevent falls.

2. Grab-bars to assist transfers should be installed in tub, showers, and toilet areas when applicable.

3. Check the water temperature with your hand before entering the tub or shower. The water temperature setting may need to be lowered.

4. A night light should be used in the bathroom if possible.

5. A bell, buzzer, or appropriate noisemaker should be placed in the bathroom for emergency use.

6. Ground fault outlets should be installed.

7. Electrical appliances should be used away from water.

8. The door lock should be a type that can be opened from the outside in an emergency.

9. Never leave a child alone in the bathtub. ***A child can drown in a few inches of water!!!***

10. If possible, locate a bathroom on the first floor.

Bibliography

Alaska Department of Health and Social Services: *Alaska Maternal and Child Health Manual for Public Health Nursing*. Alaska Department of Health and Social Services, Division of Public Health, Section of Nursing, Anchorage, Alaska; June 1994.

American Diabetes Association: *Medical Management of Pregnancy Complicated by Diabetes*. American Diabetes Association, Alexandria, Virginia; 1993.

Arkin, Elaine Bratic, and Judith E. Funkhouser: *Communicating About Alcohol and Other Drugs: Strategies for Reaching Populations at Risk*. U.S. Department of Public Health and Human Services, Rockville, Maryland; 1990.

Association of Maternal and Child Health Programs: *Caring for Mothers and Children. A Report of a Survey of FY 1987 State MCH Program Activities*. Association of Maternal and Child Health Programs, Washington, D.C.; March 1989.

Association of Maternal and Child Health Programs: *Toward the Future of Title V! A Report on Site Visits to Ten State Programs*. Association of Maternal and Child Health Programs, Washington, D.C.; November 1991.

Association of Maternal and Child Health Programs: *Meeting Needs, Building Capacities. State Perspectives on Graduate Training and Continuing Education Needs of Title V Programs*. Association of Maternal and Child Health Programs, Washington, D.C.; October 1992.

Association of Women's Health, Obstetric, and Neonatal Nurses: *Practice Resource: Preparation for Technology-Dependent Infants*. Association of Women's Health, Obstetric, and Neonatal Nurses, McLean VA; January 1993.

Bass, Alison: Few support services are available once ill children go home. *Boston Sunday Globe*, November 27, 1988.

Betz, Cecily Lynn, et al.: Altered digestive function. *Family Centered Nursing Care of Infants*, 35:1478–1480; 1994.

Block, Carol, et al.: *Home Care for High-Risk Infants, The First Year. Caring*, pp. 11–17. National Association for Home Care, Washington, D.C.; May 1989.

Boland, Mary G., and Lynn Czarniecki: Starting life with HIV, *RN*, pp. 54–58; January 1991.

Bradley, Robert, and Bettye Caldwell: Using the HOME inventory to assess the family environment. *Pediatric Nursing*, 14(2):97–102; March–April 1988.

Briggs, Nancy: Hospitals & home care: Inseparable in the '80's. *Pediatric Nursing*, 12(5):384–385; September–October 1986.

Briggs, Nancy, Connie Lierman, Julie Hazelton, Richard Wolff, Kinny Pasquera, and Elizabeth Wilson: Multidisciplinary treatment of feeding disorders in the home. *Pediatric Nursing*, 13(4):266–271; July–August 1987.

Britton, John R., and Helen Britton: Efficacy of early newborn discharge in a middle-class population. *MDC*, 138:1041–1045; November 1984.

Britton, John R., Helen Britton, and Susan Beebe: Early discharge of the term newborn: A continued dilemma. *Pediatrics*, 94(3):291–295; September 1994.

Brown, Sarah S., ed.: *Prenatal Care. Reaching Mothers. Reaching Infants*. National Academy Press, Washington, D.C.; 1988.

Boyer, D.: Prediction of postpartum depression. *NAACOG Clinical Issues in Perinatal and Women's Health Nursing*, 1(3):267–278; 1990.

Casey, Robert P.: *Investing in Our Children and Families, 1993–94 Budget Initiatives*. Executive Office, Harrisburg, Pennsylvania; 1993.

Casey, Robert P.: *Managed Competition: A Health Care System for Pennsylvania*. Report of the Pennsylvania Economic Development Partnership Health Care Committee to The Pennsylvania Economic Development Partnership. Executive Office, Harrisburg, Pennsylvania; November 1992.

Child Health Foundation: Diarrhea kills over 300 U.S. children annually. *NEWS, Child Health Foundation Newsletter*, Columbia, Maryland; June 2, 1996.

Children's Hospital of Los Angeles: *Informational Guidelines for Parents*. Children's Hospital of Los Angeles, Nutrition Support Program, Los Angeles; 1990.

Children's Hospital of Philadelphia: *Informational Guidelines for Parents*. Children's Hospital of Philadelphia, Nutrition Support Program, Philadelphia; 1991.

Commonwealth of Pennsylvania, Department of Health: *Maternal and Child Health Services*. Draft Block Grant Application, Federal Fiscal Year 1993. Pennsylvania Department of Health, Harrisburg, Pennsylvania; 1993.

Commonwealth of Pennsylvania, Department of Health: *Guide to Health Data for Pennsylvania*. State Health Data Center, Harrisburg, Pennsylvania; June 1996.

Commonwealth of Pennsylvania, Department of Public Welfare: *Pennsylvania Medical Assistance Program Eligibility Verification System Manual*. Publication 261. Pennsylvania Department of Public Welfare, Harrisburg, Pennsylvania; April 1993.

Commonwealth of Pennsylvania, Department of Public Welfare: Statistics provided by outpatient staff. Pennsylvania Department of Public Welfare, Harrisburg, Pennsylvania; May 13, 1993.

Commonwealth of Pennsylvania, Department of Public Welfare: *Overview, The Family Care Network*. Pennsylvania Department of Public Welfare, Harrisburg, Pennsylvania; 1994.

Cook, Paddy, Robert Petersen, and Dorothy Moore: *Alcohol, Tobacco, and Other Drugs May Harm the Newborn*. United States Department of Health and Human Services, Rockville, Maryland; 1990.

Cornelius, Llewellyn B.: Barriers to medical care for white, black, and Hispanic American children. *Journal of the National Medical Association*, 85(4):281–288; 1993.

Corporation for Public Broadcasting: *Miracle of Life*. Video production airing on public broadcasting series NOVA. Corporation for Public Broadcasting, Films for Humanities and Sciences, Monmouth Junction, New Jersey; 1983.

Craven, Ruth F.: *Fundamentals of Nursing*, 2nd edition. Lippincott–Raven Publishers, Philadelphia; 1996.

Cunningham, Gary, and Marshall Lindheimer: Hypertension in pregnancy. *New England Journal of Medicine*, 326(14):927–931; 1992.

Davis, Matthew, ed.: *Health Care Reform Update*, 1(8). National Association for Home Care; Washington, D.C.; May 12, 1993.

Dingell, John D., and Committee of Conference: *Conference Report, ADAMNA Reorganization Act. Title V. Home Visiting Services for At-Risk Families*. 102nd Congress, 2nd Session, House of Representatives, Report 102-546. U.S. House of Representatives, Washington, D.C.; 1994.

Donar, Mary: Community care: Pediatric home mechanical ventilation. *Holistic Nursing Practice*, 2(2):68–80; 1988.

Falkner, F., ed.: *Prevention of Infant Mortality and Morbidity. Child Health and Development*, Volume 4. Karger, Basel, Switzerland; 1985.

Farber, Anne E.: *Survey of Home Visiting Programs for Children and Families in Pennsylvania, Executive Summary*. University of Pittsburgh, University Center for Social and Urban Reseach, Office of Child Development, Pittsburgh, Pennsylvania; 1996.

Fitzgerald, Susan: 1 in 6 New mothers used cocaine, study finds. *Philadelphia Inquirer*; April 8, 1989.

Fitzgerald, Susan: How three nations shape birth. *Philadelphia Inquirer, Suburban Edition*; April 27, 1993.

Friesen, Barbara J., Joanne Griesbach, Judith Jacobs, Judith Katz-Leavy, and Dennis Olson: Improving services for families. *Children Today*, pp. 18–22; July–August 1988.

Federal Register: Medicare regulations. *Federal Register: Rules and Regulations*, 54(153); August 14, 1989.

Fleming, Barbara W.: Assessing and promoting positive parenting in adolescent mothers. *MCN*, 18:32–37; January–February 1993.

Grabert, B., C. Wardell, and S. Harburg: Home phototherapy. *Clinical Pediatrics*, 25:291–294; 1986.

Harrison, H., and A. Kositsky: *The Premature Baby Book*. St. Martin's Press, New York; 1983.

Henrikson, Mary, Ginna Wall, Dona Lethbridge, and Vicki McClurg: Nursing diagnosis and obstetric, gynecologic, and neonatal nursing: Breastfeeding as an example. *JOGN Thoughts and Opinions*, 21(6); November–December 1992.

Herman, Robin: France wants me to have this baby. *Washington Post*; May 1, 1990.

Hoerlin, Bettina Yaffe: *Targeting for the Future: Health Care in the Philadelphia Region*. Report to The Pew Charitable Trusts, Philadelphia, Pennsylvania; January 1989.

Howard, Tracy: *Kids Ending Hunger. What Can We Do?* Andrews and McMeel, A Universal Press Syndicate Co., Kansas City, Missouri; 1992.

Hyde-Robertson, Barbara L.: The necessity for maternal–infant perinatal home care. *Caring*, pp. 26–31. National Association for Home Care, Washington, D.C.; December 1992.

Infante-Rivard, Claire, Gisele Filion, Mona Baumgarten, Madeleine Bourassa, Johanne Labelle, and Monique Messier: A public health home intervention among families of low socioeconomic status. *CHC*, 18(2):102; Spring 1989.

Institute of Medicine: *Nutrition During Pregnancy and Lactation*. National Academy Press, Washington, D.C.; 1990.

Johns Hopkins Oral Rehydration Project: *Outpatient Oral Rehydration Therapy Protocol*. Johns Hopkins Oral Rehydration Project, Baltimore, Maryland; 1991.

Johnson, S., and D. Kraut: *Pregnancy and Bedrest: A Guide for the Pregnant Woman and Her Family*. St. Martin's Press, New York; 1990.

Langevin, Jeanne: Using home health aids in a high-risk infant program. *Caring*, pp. 40–43. National Association for Home Care, Washington, D.C.; June 1988.

Marecki, Marsha: Postpartum followup goals and assessment. *JOGN*, pp. 214–218; August 1979.

Marks, Margaret G.: *Introductory Pediatric Nursing*, 4th edition. Lippincott–Raven Publishers, Philadelphia; 1994.

McAnarney, Elizabeth R.: Experience with an adolescent health care program. *Public Health Reports*, 90(5):412–416; September–October 1975.

McAnarney, Elizabeth R.: Development of an adolescent maternity project in Rochester, New York. *Public Health Reports*, 92(2):154–159; March–April 1977.

NAACOG: *Criteria Established for Identifying At-Risk Infants*, 14(10). NAACOG, Washington, D.C.; October 1987.

NAACOG: *OGN Nursing Practice Resource: Neonatal Skin Care*. NAACOG, Washington, D.C.; 1992.

National Center for Education in Maternal and Child Health: *Reaching Out: A Directory of National Organizations Related to Maternal and Child Health*. National Center for Education in Maternal and Child Health, Washington, D.C.; March 1989.

Nettina, Sandra M.: *Lippincott Manual of Nursing Practice*, 6th edition. Lippincott–Raven Publishers, Philadelphia; 1996.

North Carolina Department of Health: *MCH Manual*. Department of Public Health, Durham, North Carolina; 1992.

Nuttal, P.: Maternal responses to home apnea monitoring of infants. *Nursing Research*, 37:354–357; 1988.

Oehler, Jerri N., et al.: How to target infants at highest risk for developmental delay. *Maternal–Child Nursing*, 18:20–23; January–February 1993.

Olds, D.: The prenatal/infancy project: A strategy for responding to the needs of high risk mothers and their children. *Prevention in Human Services*, 7(1):59–87; 1989.

Olds, D., C. Henderson, R. Tatlebaum, and R. Chamberlin: Improving the delivery of prenatal care and outcomes of pregnancy: A randomized trial of nurse home visitation. *Pediatrics*, 77(1):16–28; January 1986.

Olds, D., and H. Kitzman: Can home visitation improve the health of women and children at environmental risk? *Pediatrics*, 1(1):108–116; July 1990.

Pennsylvania Department of Health: *Block Grant, Commonwealth of Pennsylvania Preventive and Primary Care Services for Pregnant Women, Mothers, and Infants up to Age 1, Component A*, p. 64. Pennsylvania Department of Health, Division of Maternal Child Health, Harrisburg, Pennsylvania.

Pennsylvania Department of Health: *Vital Statistics 1990*. Pennsylvania Department of Health, State Health Data Center, Harrisburg, Pennsylvania; 1992.

Pennsylvania Healthy Mothers, Healthy Babies Coalition: *Pennsylvania Healthy Mothers, Healthy Babies Coalition* Pennsylvania Healthy Mothers, Healthy Babies Coalition, Bryn Mawr, Pennsylvania; 1992.

Pennsylvania Partnerships for Children: *Our Children, Our Future.* Breakfast on Children's Health Issues. Pennsylvania Partnerships for Children, Harrisburg, Pennsylvania; October 9, 1991.

Pennsylvania Partnerships for Children: *Kids Count.* State Grant Proposal for Pennsylvania. Pennsylvania Partnerships for Children, Harrisburg, Pennsylvania; August 13, 1992.

Perrin, James M.: Chronically ill children, in America, the case for home care. *Journal for Physicians in Home Care*; Spring 1987.

Philadelphia Department of Public Health: *Selected Resident Birth and Death Data by Health District, by Census Tract and by Neighborhood, 1983–1993.* Department of Public Health, Philadelphia, 1994.

Reece, S.: Social support and the early maternal experience for primiparas over 35. *Maternal–Child Nursing Journal,* 3:91–98; July–September 1993.

Reeder, S., L. Martin, and D. Koniak-Griffin: *Maternity Nursing, Family Newborn and Women's Health Care,* 18th edition. Lippincott–Raven Publishers, Philadelphia; 1997.

Richmond, Frederick, Martha Wade Steketee, et al.: *The State of the Child: A Profile of Pennsylvania's Children.* Waldman Graphics, Philadelphia; 1993.

Roberts, Joyce: Current perspectives in preeclampsia. *Journal of Nurse Midwifery,* 39(2):70–90; 1994.

Rogatz, Peter: Perspective on home care. *Public Health Nursing,* 4(1):7–8; March 1987.

Rosen, C., D. Glaze, and J. Frost: Home monitor followup of persistent apnea and bradycardia in preterm infants. *American Journal of Diseases in Children,* 140:547–550; 1986.

Shelton, Terri I., Elizabeth Jeppson, and Beverly Johnson: *Family Centered Care for Children with Special Health Care Needs,* 2nd edition. Association for the Care of Children's Health, U.S. Public Health Service, Division of Maternal Child Health, Rockville, Maryland; 1987.

Sills, Joanne: Infant deaths soar in areas. *Philadelphia Daily News*; July 8, 1992.

Sirkka, L.: Health promotion in child and family health care: The role of the Finnish public health nurses. *Public Health Nursing,* 11(1):32–37; February 1994.

Smith, Judy: The dangers of prenatal cocaine use. *Maternal–Child Nursing,* 13:174–179; May–June 1992.

South Carolina Department of Health and Environmental Control: *Comprehensive Risk Screening for Patient Referrals.* South Carolina Department of Health and Environmental Control, Maternal Health, Columbia, South Carolina; October 1992.

Stanwick, Richard S., Michael E. K. Moffat, Yvonne Robitaille, Aline Edmond, and Caroline Dok: An evaluation of the routine postnatal public health nurse home visit. *Canadian Journal of Public Health,* 73:200–205; May–June 1982.

Starn, J.: Community health nursing visits for at risk women and infants. *Journal of Community Health Nursing,* 9(2):103–110; 1992.

Streeter, N. S.: Discharge planning home care. *Journal of Perinatal and Neonatal Nursing* 5(1); 1991.

Sullivan, Joan, et al.: Can we help the substance abusing mother and infant? *Maternal–Child Nursing,* 18:153–157; May–June 1993.

United Way of Pennsylvania: *Report of the Success-By-Six Coalition: Helping All Children Succeed for Life.* United Way of Pennsylvania, Harrisburg, Pennsylvania; June 1992.

U.S.D.L., Occupational Safety and Health, Office of Health Compliance Assistance: *OSHA Instruction CPL 2-2, 44A,* p. 4. U.S. Department of Labor Occupational Safety and Health, Office of Health Compliance Assistance, Washington, D.C.; August 15, 1988.

U.S.D.P.H., Agency for Health Care Policy and Research: *The 50 Most Frequent Diagnosis-Related Groups (DRO's), Diagnoses, and Procedures: Statistics by Hospital Size and Location.* Hospital Studies Program Research Note 13. U.S. Department of Public Health, Agency for Health Care Policy and Research, Rockville, Maryland; September 1990.

U.S.D.P.H., Agency for Health Care Policy and Research: *Research Activities: Contracts Awarded for Low Birthweight, Health Care for Women, Barriers to Quality Care Persist.* Publication No. 158. U.S. Department of Public Health, Agency for Health Care Policy and Research, Rockville, Maryland; November 1992.

U.S.D.P.H., Agency for Health Care Policy and Research: *Research Activities: Number of Uninsured Children on the Rise, Less than 15 Percent of America's Health Care Dollar Spent on Children.* Publication No. 162. U.S. Department of Public Health, Agency for Health Care Policy and Research, Rockville, Maryland; March 1993.

U.S.D.P.H., Agency for Health Care Policy and Research: *Research Activities: Women Planning Pregnancy*

Often Switch to HMO's. Publication No. 163. U.S. Department of Public Health, Agency for Health Care Policy and Research, Rockville, Maryland; April 1993.

U.S.D.P.H., Agency for Health Care Policy and Research: *Research Activities: Uninsured Patients More Likely to Die Prematurely*. Publication No. 169. U.S. Department of Public Health, Agency for Health Care Policy and Research, Rockville, Maryland; October 1993.

U.S.D.P.H., Agency for Health Care Policy and Research: *Research Activities: Financially Troubled Hospitals Face Difficult Choices, Outlook Poor for Very Young Babies with AIDS, Teen Health Programs Often Deficient in On Site Services*. Publication No. 170. U.S. Department of Public Health, Agency for Health Care Policy and Research, Rockville, Maryland; November 1993.

U.S.D.P.H.H.S.: *Caring for Our Future: The Content of Prenatal Care*. U.S. Department of Public Health and Human Services, Washington, D.C.; 1989.

U.S.P.H.S.: *Back to Sleep: Reducing the Risk of Sudden Infant Death Syndrome—What You Can Do*. The American Academy of Pediatrics, SIDS Alliance,, and the Association of SIDS Program Professionals. U.S. Public Health Service, Washington, D.C.

Vrazo, Fawn: Pregnant doctors in distress. *Philadeinhia Inquirer*; February 17, 1990.

Vrazo, Fawn: Lying in is now out for many new mothers. *Philadelphia Inquirer*; August 17, 1990.

Vrazo, Fawn: Lying in is out as insurers cut post-childbirth coverage. *Philadelphia Inquirer*; August 7, 1993.

Wasik, B., D. Bryant, and C. Lyons: *Home Visiting: Procedures for Helping Families*. Sage Publications, Newbury Park, California; 1990.

Weston, Donna R., Barbara Ivins, Barry Zuckerman, Coryl Jones, and Richard Lopez: *Drug Exposed Babies: Research and Clinical Issues*. National Center for Clinical Infant Programs, Washington, D.C.; June 1989.

Williams, Lenore, and Mary Cooper: Nurse managed postpartum home care. *JOGN Principles and Practice*, pp. 25–31; January–February 1993.

Wisconsin Association for Perinatal Care: *Early Discharge—Short Term Length of Stay*. Wisconsin Association for Perinatal Care; June 1993.

Yariover, Mark J., Deloras Jones, and Michael D. Miller: Perinatal care of low risk mothers and infants. *New England Journal of Medicine*, 294(13):702–705; March 25, 1976.

Young, L., D. Creighton, and R. Sauve: The needs of families of infants discharged home with continous oxygen therapy. *Journal of Obstetric, Gynecolgic, and Neonatal Nursing*, 17:187–193; 1987.

Zuravin, Susan J.: *Child Maltreatment and Teenage First Births: A Relationship Mediated by Chronic Sociodemographic Stress?* American Orthopsychiatric Association, Washington, D.C.; January 1988.

Additional Resources

Free or low-cost educational material can be obtained from the following additional health information resources.

U.S. Department of Health and Human Services
Public Health Service Office of Disease Prevention and Health Promotion
ONHIC, P.O. Box 1133
Washington, DC 20013-1133
(800) 336-4797
Request the *Health Information Resources Catalogue*

Maternal Child Health Bureau
March of Dimes Birth Defects Foundation
National Center for Education in Maternal Child Health
Write to: National Maternal Child Health Clearing House
8201 Greensboro Drive, Suite 600
McLean, VA 22102
(703) 821-8955, ext. 254 or 265
Request *Prenatal Care, A Resource Guide*

Appendices

The appendices of this manual contain additional information that the provider will find helpful in creating a well-organized Maternal–Newborn Home Health Program. *Section 1* contains clinical records designed for a Maternal–Newborn Home Health Visiting Program that also seeks Medicare certification or accreditation through JCAHO or NLN. Included is a copy of the standard Plan of Care developed for use by the Health Care Financing Administration (HCFA; *Appendix A*). This document records the physician orders for home care services and should be completed by the nurse. Also included are clinical records to be used by the nurse in developing a comprehensive plan of nursing care, but which would also be of use to professionals in other disciplines such as physical therapy and social work. Included in addition to the HCFA form are the following.

1. **Home Health Client Rights and Consent Forms:** Organizations will want to modify this form to assure that clients have the hotline phone number to their individual state surveyor office. For Medicare-certified agencies, allowing clients access to this number is a federal requirement. *(See Appendices B–D.)*
2. **Postpartum/Infant Universal Assessment Form:** Many states now recognize the need to provide for a least one home visit to postpartum women and infants discharged from the hospital 24–48 hours postdelivery. Some states have gone as far as mandating at least one home visit by law. Few insurers, hopefully, would argue the need to provide at least one home visit if not a series of visits to an infant detained for treatment in a special care nursery. As nurses, we need to advocate in our fight against infant mortality for the provision of at least one postpartum/infant home visit for all families. The home is where the infant's day-to-day care is provided. Without inclusion of the home environment, a comprehensive risk assessment will not be complete. Much of the tragedy of infant mortality can be prevented if we are aware of problems and can address them where the child lives.

   This form is used on the very first visit made by the nurse and is used for all mothers and infants whether or not they had a healthy or complicated delivery and recovery. *(See Appendix E.)*
3. **Initial Evaluation Form:** This is to be completed by the nurse as part of the medical assessment for newborns admitted to home care after the first postpartum/infant universal assessment. These are newborns who will receive visits according to a prescribed Plan of Care done on the enclosed HCFA form. *(See Appendix F.)*
4. **Current Medication Profile:** This is to be completed by the nurse at the first visit and updated at each subsequent visit. The nurse should always review side effects and contraindications in addition to always verifying the medicaton orders with the prescriptions obtained from the pharmacy. The nurse should never assume that the parents are calculating dosages correctly, and should observe them at least once as they perform these procedures. Although aides do not administer medications, they should be oriented to this in order to be more familiar with the client's needs. *(See Appendix G.)*
5. **Nursing Plan of Care and Progress Record:** This is to be used by the nurse for subsequent home visits. *(See Appendix H.)*
6. **Nursing Progress Notes:** This is for use by nurses and aides. Home health aides should summarize care each visit or shift. *(See Appendix I.)*

7. **Pediatric Intake and Output:** A clinical record tool the nurse may find helpful to have the client's family and the aide maintain. It should be reviewed by the nurse on each visit. *(See Appendix J.)*
8. **Home Needs Assessment Form:** This tool is not a required, but is helpful in obtaining additional information about the homes of children whose care requires technological support. Prior to hospital discharge, questions such as "Does the child's home have adequate electrical resources to support the needed equipment?" should be addressed. Nurses can also use this form to provide a prehospital discharge visit to the home for an infant with medical technology needs. *(See Appendix K.)*
9. **Discharge Summary:** This is to be completed by the nurse at the end of care. *(See Appendix L.)*

Appendices M–R provide the user with forms that will be helpful in evaluating the program for effectiveness. The Case Management Log is recommended for use with infants admitted to home care after the first universal home visit. *(See Appendix M.)* Completion of the log is necessary for infants admitted to the high-risk infant follow-up program, which recommends that regularly scheduled home visits be made throughout the first year for infants with significant social and or medical problems. *Appendices N–R* contain forms that will be helpful in maintaining and evaluating qualitative and quantitative data.

The Bibliography preceding the appendices will be useful in developing a resource library. The manual concludes with a list of abbreviations, a helpful glossary, and a detailed index.

Appendix A

Department of Health and Human Services
Health Care Financing Administration

Form Approved
OMB No. 0938-0357

HOME HEALTH CERTIFICATION AND PLAN OF TREATMENT

1. Patient's HI Claim No.	2. SOC Date	3. Certification Period From: To:	4. Medical Record No.	5. Provider No.

6. Patient's Name and Address	7. Provider's Name and Address

8. Date of Birth:	9. Sex ☐ M ☐ F	10. Medications: Dose/Frequency/Route (N)ew (C)hanged
11. ICD-9-CM	Principal Diagnosis	Date
12. ICD-9-CM	Surgical Procedure	Date
13. ICD-9-CM	Other Pertinent Diagnoses	Date

14. DME and Supplies	15. Safety Measures:
16. Nutritional Req.	17. Allergies:

18.A. Functional Limitations

1 ☐ Amputation
2 ☐ Bowel/Bladder (Incontinence)
3 ☐ Contracture
4 ☐ Hearing
5 ☐ Paralysis
6 ☐ Endurance
7 ☐ Ambulation
8 ☐ Speech
9 ☐ Legally Blind
A ☐ Dyspnea with Minimal Exertion
B ☐ Other (Specify)

18.B. Activities Permitted

1 ☐ Complete Bedrest
2 ☐ Bedrest BRP
3 ☐ Up as Tolerated
4 ☐ Transfer Bed/Chair
5 ☐ Exercises Prescribed
6 ☐ Partial Weight Bearing
7 ☐ Independent at Home
8 ☐ Crutches
9 ☐ Cane
A ☐ Wheelchair
B ☐ Walker
C ☐ No Restrictions
D ☐ Other (Specify)

19. Mental Status: 1 ☐ Oriented 2 ☐ Comatose 3 ☐ Forgetful 4 ☐ Depressed 5 ☐ Disoriented 6 ☐ Lethargic 7 ☐ Agitated 8 ☐ Other

20. Prognosis: 1 ☐ Poor 2 ☐ Guarded 3 ☐ Fair 4 ☐ Good 5 ☐ Excellent

21. Orders for Discipline and Treatments (Specify Amount/Frequency/Duration)

22. Goals/Rehabilitation Potential/Discharge Plans

23. Verbal Start of Care and Nurse's Signature and Date Where Applicable:

24. Physician's Name and Address

25. Date HHA received Signed POT

26. I ☐ certify ☐ recertify that the above home health services are required and are authorized by me with a written plan for treatment which will be periodically reviewed by me. This patient is under my care, is confined to his home, and is in need of intermittent skilled nursing care and/or physical or speech therapy or has been furnished home health services based on such a need and no longer has a need for such care or therapy, but continues to need occupational therapy.

27. Attending Physician's Signature (required on 485 Kept on File in Medical Records of HHA)

Date Signed

Consent for Treatment, Release of Information, Assignment of Benefits, Notice of Client Rights

Client Name: ______________________________

Address: ______________________________

City: ____________________ State: ________ Zip: ____________

I, ______________________ (custodial parent or legal guardian), ____________ (relationship) of ____________ (minor client) intending to be legally bound, hereby:

1. Consent to such care and treatment by ______________________, and its employees and agents (collectively, the "Agency"), as prescribed by the client's physician or dictated by the client's condition.
2. Authorize the Agency to release any medical records in its possession concerning the client as may be required by law or to pay benefits on the client's behalf. I authorize the client's physicians, insurers, and hospitals to release such medical records to the Agency at the Agency's request.
3. Authorize my insurer to disclose to the Agency the terms and extent of my coverage, and the amount of payments made to me for services provided by the Agency.
4. Assign, transfer, and set over to the Agency all of my or the client's rights to insurance proceeds or other funds to which I am or the client is or will become entitled as a result of the services rendered by the Agency.
5. Consent to and authorize payment, which would otherwise be payable to me or the client, to be made directly to the Agency. The Agency may issue a receipt for such payment which shall discharge the insurance company of its obligations under the policy to the extent of such payment.
6. Agree that I remain individually responsible to pay the Agency for all charges not paid for any reason by the insurer or other third-party payor. I understand that payment in full is due upon receipt of my bill. If payment for the Agency's services is made directly to me by my insurer, I agree to endorse the check to the provider and forward it to the Agency within three days of receipt.

A photocopy of this document, if executed, shall be considered as effective and valid as the original.

The effect of this form and the Client's Rights and Responsibilities on the back of this form have been explained to me by the Agency and I understand its content and significance.

Date: ____________ Signature: ______________________

Name: ______________________
(please print)

Appendix C

Home Health Care Client's Bill of Rights/Responsibilities

As a home health care client you have the right to:

1. Standard: Right to be informed and to participate in planning care and treatment (1) The client has the right to be informed in advance about the care to be furnished.

2. Be given information about your rights and responsibilities for receiving home health care services, in terms and language you can reasonably expect to understand.

3. Receive a timely response from the Home Health Care Agency regarding your request for home health care services.

4. Be given information of the Home Health Care Agency charges and policy concerning payment for services, including your eligibility for third party reimbursement.

5. Choose your home health care providers.

6. Be given appropriate and professional quality home health care services without discrimination against your race, creed, color, religion, sex, national origin, sexual preference, handicap, or age.

7. The client's family or guardian may exercise the client's rights when the client has been judged incompetent.

8. The HHA must investigate complaints made by a client or the client's family or guardian regarding treatment or care that is (or fails to be) furnished, or regarding the lack of respect for the client's property by anyone furnishing services on behalf of the HHA, and must document both the existence of the complaint and the resolution of the complaint.

9. Be treated with courtesy and respect by all who provide home health care services to you; to have your property treated with respect.

10. Before the care is initiated, the HHA must inform the client, orally and in writing, of
    a. The extent of which payment may be expected from Medicare, Medicaid, or any other federally funded or aided program known to the HHA
    b. The charges for services that will not be covered by Medicare; and
    c. The charges that the individual may have to pay
    d. The client has the right to be advised orally and in writing of any changes in payment from last financial counseling.

11. The client has the right to be advised orally and in writing of any changes in payment. The HHA must advise the client of these changes orally and in writing as soon as possible, but no later than 15 working days from the date that the HHA becomes aware of a change.

12. Be given the necessary information so you will be able to give informed consent for your treatment prior to the start of any treatment.

13. Participate in the development of your home health care plan, to be informed in advance about the care to be provided and any changes in the care to be provided, including anticipated transfer of your care to another health care facility and/or termination of home health care service.

14. To be advised in advance of the disciplines that will provide care, and the frequency of visits proposed to be provided.

15. Be given data privacy and confidentiality; review your clinical record at your request.

16. Voice grievances regarding treatment or care that is (or fails to be) furnished, or regarding any lack of respect for privacy by anyone who is furnishing services on behalf of the home health care agency, without being subject to discrimination or reprisal for doing so.

    * Call ____________________ to voice a grievance and/or recommend changes in policies or services.
    * Medicare/Medicaid clients may also call a Hotline # (1-800-222-0989) to report grievances from 8:30 am–5:00 pm with answering service for non-business hours. This is *not* the number to reach the Home Health Care Agency or to obtain Medicare coverage/billing information.

17. Refuse all or part of your care to the extent permitted by law; to be informed of the expected consequences of such action.

18. The client's family or guardian may exercise the client's rights when the client has been judged incompetent.

Appendix D

Client Responsibilities

As a home health care client you have the responsibility to:

1. Give accurate and complete health information concerning your past illnesses, hospitalizations, medications, allergies, and other pertinent items.
2. Assist in developing and maintaining a safe environment.
3. Inform the Home Health Care Agency when you will not be able to keep a home health care visit.
4. Participate in the development and update of your home health care plan.
5. Adhere to your developed/updated home health care plan.
6. Request further information concerning anything you do not understand.
7. Give information regarding concerns and problems you have to Home Health Care Agency staff member.

Advance Directives

An advance directive is a written instruction, such as a living will or durable power of attorney for health care, recognized under state law, relating to the provision of health care when an individual's condition makes him/her unable to express his/her wishes. The intent of these provisions is to enhance an individual's control over medical treatment decisions.

The Agency's policy regarding implementation of a client's advance directive is to comply to the best of its ability with those instructions.

1. The client has been informed of the state living will law. Yes _____ No _____
2. Does the client have a living will? Yes _____ No _____
3. If so, is there a copy of the advance directive in the client's medical record? Yes _____ No _____

Client Signature: ______________________________ Date: ________________

Appendix E

Postpartum/Infant Universal Home Risk Assessment Form

Mother's Name: ______________________ Date of Birth: ____________

Address: ______________________________________ Phone: (   ) ____________

Language: ______ Race: ____ Marital Status: ____ Education Level: ____

Emergency Contact: ______________________ Phone: (   ) ____________

Infant's Name: ______________________ Date of Birth: ____________ Gest. age in wks.: ____

vag.: ____ VBAC: ____ prim. C/S: ____ rep. C/S: ____ forceps: ____ vac.: ____ vag.: ____ BW: ____

Does infant have temporary eligibility card? Yes ___ No ___ Has patient notified caseworker of birth? Yes ___ No ___

Ins. type: ____________ Ins. No.: ____________ Mother's SS No.: ____________

Has patient been informed of insurance benefits MA/HMO? Yes ____ No ____

Current Medications: ______________________ Hospital of delivery: ______________________

			ABNORMAL		
MOTHER ASSESSMENT		NORMAL	FAJ MD	FAJ / Home Care Provider	COMMENTS
SKIN					
METABOLIC	TPR				
NEURO					
HEENT					
CARDIOVASC.	BP				
CHEST	Lungs/Breasts				
MUSCULO/ SKELETAL	Upper/ Lower extremities				
GI	Nutrition/Elimination				
GU	Voiding, Locia, Fundus				
INFANT ASSESSMENT					
SKIN	Color/Cond./Cord				
METABOLIC	TPR				
NEURO	Sleeping/Activity reflexes/Suck				
	Fontanelles				
HEENT	Auditory/ Visual response				
CARDIOVASC.	Apical pulse				
CHEST	Lungs				
MUSCULO/ SKELETAL	Muscle tone				
GI	Feeding tye/Amt/Freq. Elimination				
GU	Genitalia/Anus Voiding				

COMPLICATIONS OF LABOR AND/OR DELIVERY (Check all that apply)

____ None known
____ Febrile (>100 or 39°C) or labor >20 hr.
____ Meconium
____ Premature rupture of membrane (>12 hrs)
____ Del. <37 wks.
____ Seizure during preg. or labor
____ Precipitous labor (<3 hrs.)
____ Cephalopelvic disproportion
____ Abruptio placenta or other causes of bleeding
____ Fetal distress
____ Dysfunctional labor
____ Breech/malpresentation
____ Other—specify: ____________________

RISK ASSESSMENT (circle risk score if applicable)

I. Life Transitions

2 Denial/rejection re: pregnancy
1 Hx current/recent incest/rape victim
1 Hx infant/child chronic disability
1 Hx of fetal death/other inf./preg. loss
1 Adoption/termination considered
1 Suspected domestic violence

II. Emotional Status

1 Hx of mental illness/mental health treat./hosp.
1 Unresolved grief/signif. loss
2 Suicidal ideation
1 Feels isolation/alone/inadeq. support system
1 Questionable coping
1 Hx of postpartum depression
1 Evidence of low self-esteem

III. Substance Abuse/Risk-Taking Behaviors

3 Current/recent abuse of alcohol
3 Current/recent abuse of street drugs
3 Current/recent abuse of presc. meds
1 Law enforcement involvement
1 Sexual risk-taking behaviors
1 Tobacco use or 2nd-hand smoke exposure

IV. Parenting issues (observed/expressed)

1 Teen/inexperienced parent
1 Develop. issues (child/fam. expectations)
1 Discipline issues
1 Relationship issues (bond/nurturing)
1 Hx child abuse/neglect, now resolved
2 Child abuse/neglect, current
1 3 Or more children < 6 yrs. of age

V. Educational/Cultural Factors

1 Low literacy/limited intellectual ability
1 Cognitive deficits
1 Language barriers
1 Ed. level l2th or less
2 Ed. level 10th or less
3 Ed. level 9th or less or < 17 y.o.
1 Culture/Beliefs

VI. Economic/Resource Needs

1 Insuff. income to meet basic needs
1 No transportation
2 Inadequate food
1 Legal needs
2 Chronic difficulty accessing "system"
1 Child care problems
1 Medicaid problems

VII. A. Medical/Nutritional Factors

2 Abnl. phys. fndgs. this assess.
1 Problems w/chosen FP method
1 Short interconceptual period (<1 yr)
1 Grand multigravida (>7 preg.)
2 Anemia mother < 10.8
2 chronic disease
3 HIV/AIDS
2 Problem initiating breastfeeding
1 PICA
1 Anorexia/bulemia/fad diets

VII. B. Medical/Nutritional Factors

2 Abnl. phys. fndgs. this assess.
3 Prenatal exp. to drugs/alcohol
2 Anemia infant
1 Failure to thrive in sibs., prev. or existing
2 Dx or suspected malabsorption
2 Symptoms of intolerance to formula
2 Infant diarrhea
2 GE reflux
2 Low birth weight infant < 2500 gm
3 Low birth weight infant < 1500 gm

2 Problem establishing breastfeeding
3 Inadequate prenatal. care
__ initiated 1st trimester
__ initiated 2nd trimester
__ initiated 3rd trimester
1 Previous hosp. of sibs. in 1 st yr.
3 Extended NICU hospitalization
2 Medical problems r/t prematurity
2 Medical problems r/t congenital anomalies
2 STD exp. in preg., untreated
1 Lead exposure

VIII. Environmental

1 Housing
1 Utilities
1 Refrigeration
1 Water/sewer
1 High risk/unsafe neighborhood
1 Inadeq. prep. for infant

SUMMARY OF ASSESSMENT AND RISK FACTORS: ____________________

REFERRALS/PLAN	DATE OF APPT.	CONTACT PERSON/PROVIDER	PHONE
Postpartum Exam			
WIC			
Pediatrician/PCP			
MA Caseworker			
Other			

EVALUATION

_____ Discharge to primary, no further HC required
_____ Open to home care follow/up
_____ Meets high risk admission criteria

EPSDT: _____ yes _____ no
PCP name: ____________________
Address: ____________________

NRSG INTERVENTIONS/TEACHING	DONE	DEFERRED TO HC	EVALUATION (response to teaching)
Postpartum Care			
Feeding			
Bathing/Skin/Cord Care			
Infection Control			
Safety (home/car)			
S/S illness/Taking Temperature			

Nurse signature: ____________________ Date: __________

Appendix F

Initial Evaluation Form

Client Name: ______________________ Date of Birth: ____________

Address: ______________________ Phone: ( ) ____________

Primary Physician: ______________________

Physician Address: ______________________ Phone: ( ) ____________

Primary Diagnosis: ______________ Secondary Diagnosis: ______________

Allergies: ______________ Functional Limitations: ______________

Client's Primary Caregiver: ______________________ Relationship: ____________

PHYSICAL ASSESSMENT		NORM.	ABNORM.	DESCRIBE/MEASURE/PAST MEDICAL HISTORY
SKIN	Color			
	Condition/Turgor			
METABOLIC	Temperature			
NEURO	Mental Status/ Headaches/Blackouts			
	Activity/Gait			
	Pupils			
	Seizures			
HEENT	Appearance			
	Neck Mobility			
	Lymph Nodes			
CARDIO-VASCULAR	Apical Pulse			
	Peripheral Pulse			
	Blood Pressure			
	Circulation/Capillary Refill			
CHEST	Configuration/Circumference			
	Auscultation			
	Respiration/Rate			
PSYCHO-SOCIAL	Interactions			
	Affect			
	Developmental Milestones			
MUSCULO/ SKELETAL	Upper Extremities			
	Lower Extremities			
ABDOMEN	Shape			
	Bowel Sounds			
	Palpation			
GU	Voiding			
	BM			

RN Signature: ______________________ License #: ____________ Date: ________

Client Name: ______________________

NUTRITIONAL STATUS	PO/Enteral	
	Parenteral	
	Feeding Issues	Weight

SAFETY ASSESSMENT	YES	NO	COMMENTS
Teaching: Basic Home Safety?			
CPR Training Reviewed/Reinforced?			
Reviewed plan for emergency medical situation/emergency phone numbers?			
Is "do not resuscitate" order applicable?			If yes, signed order must be in clinical record
Reviewed safety instruction related to equipment and care being provided?			
Physical/psychosocial environment adequate for patient care?			

Other medical personnel providing care (specify name and phone): ______________________

List equipment in home/specify instructions for use given: ______________________

Reason for visit/home care needs: ______________________

Nursing diagnosis(es): ______________________

Short-term goal(s): ______________________

Long-term goal(s): ______________________

Nursing interventions (treatment, teaching, etc.): ______________________

Evaluation (response to interventions): ______________________

Referrals: ______________________

Date and Nursing Care Plan for next visit: ______________________

Communication to M.D./Agency Office/Other: ______________________

Change in orders/Change in medication: ______________________

(specify change and attach completed physician verbal order form)

RN Signature: ______________________ License #: ____________ Date: ________

Current Medication Profile

Client Name: ______________________ Allergies: ______________________

MEDICATION (Dose, Frequency, Rate)	MODIFICATION SINCE DATE OF REFERRAL	PURPOSE	SIGNIFICANT SIDE EFFECTS	INSTRUCTION *	UNDERSTANDING **

PHARMACY: PHONE:

* INSTRUCTION CODES:
1—Verbal Instructions given
2—Medication Sheet left in home
3—Medication Sheet & verbal instructions given
4—Side effects/adverse reactions reviewed
5—Dose & frequency reviewed
6—Purpose instructed
7—All of the above

** G—Good F—Fair P—Poor

Appendix **H**

Nursing Plan of Care and Progress Record

CLIENT NAME: ______________________________

ADDRESS: ______________________________

____

____

PHONE: (   ) ______________________________

ALLERGIES: ______________________________

HHA Supervisory Visit	Yes ____	No ____
PT satisfied with care?	Yes ____	No ____
HHA Following Care Plan	Yes ____	No ____
Care plan updated?	Yes ____	No ____

HHA's name ______________________________

LEAD SCREENING STATUS
1. Is infant the appropriate age for lead screening? Yes ____ No ____
2. If yes, does caregiver know if it was done? Yes ____ No ____
3. Does caregiver know results? Yes ____ No ____

IMMUNIZATION STATUS
1. Did infant receive any immunizations at last visit? Yes ____ No ____
2. Has infant received any immunizations since birth? Yes ____ No ____
3. If yes, when and which ones? (if changed from last visit): ______________________________
   Name of last pediatric provider: ______________________________
4. Is infant appropriately immunized (as reported by caregiver)? Yes ____ No ____
5. If no, why? (as explained by caregiver): ______________________________

Date of last appt.: ________ Date of next appt.: ________

SKILLED OBSERVATION/ASSESSMENT

	Normal	Abnormal	Describe		Normal	Abnormal	Describe
Metabolic (TPR)				Genitourinary			
HEENT				Musculoskeletal			
Cardiovascular				Neurological			
Respiratory				Integumentary			
ABD/G.I.				Psychosocial			
Nutrition/Wt.				Other			

Medical Diagnosis: ______________________________

Reason for Visit/Homecare Needs: ______________________________

Nursing Diagnosis(es): ______________________________

Short-Term Goal(s): ______________________________

Long-Term Goal(s): ______________________________

Nursing Interventions (treatment, teaching, etc.): ______________________________

____

____

Evaluation (response to interventions): ______________________________

____

____

Date and Nursing Care Plan for next visit: ______________________________

____

Communication to M.D./Agency Office/Other: ______________________________

Changes in orders/changes in medication: ______________________________

(specify change and attach completed verbal order form)

RN Signature: ______________________________ License #: ________________ Date: ____________

Nursing Progress Notes

Client Name: ______________________________

DATE	

Appendix J

Pediatric Intake and Output Record for Parents' Use

Client Name: ______________________________

	Date/Day	Feeding Amt & Time	Amt & Time	Amt & Time	Amt & Time	Amt & Time	Amt & Time	Amt & Time	Total # of Feedings/ per day	Wet Diapers (Mark with X for each change)	Total # of wet diapers/day (void/cc)	BM
MONDAY												
TUESDAY												
WEDNESDAY												
THURSDAY												
FRIDAY												
SATURDAY												
SUNDAY												
MONDAY												
TUESDAY												
WEDNESDAY												
THURSDAY												
FRIDAY												
SATURDAY												
SUNDAY												

Home Care Needs Assessment Tool

CLIENT

Name: ______________________ Client's DOB: ______________ Client's Age: ________

Client's Ins. #: ______________________ Clients SS#: ______________________

Client's Race: ______________ Client's Sex: ________

Current Telephone #: (   ) ______________ Current Telephone #: (   ) ______________

INSTITUTION: ______________________

_____ Home _____ Shelter _____ Homeless _____ Staying with Relatives

Address: ____
(street (apt.) (City) (Zip)

EMERGENCY CONTACT PERSONS

Name: ______________________ Relationship: ______________ Age: ________

Phone: ______________

Address: ____
(street (apt.) (City) (Zip)

MOTHER'S DATA

Name: ______________________ Phone: ______________ Age: ______________

Address: ____
(street (apt.) (City) (Zip)

Best Time to Contact: ______________________

FATHER'S DATA

Name: ______________________ Phone: ______________ Age: ______________

Address: ____
(street (apt.) (City) (Zip)

Best Time to Contact: ______________________

CHILD'S DOCTOR (must use PCP if applicable)

Name: ______________________ Hospital: ______________ Phone: __________

Address: ____
(street (apt.) (City) (Zip)

CONSULTING DOCTORS ON CARE

1. ______________________ (Name) ______________ (Phone)
2. ______________________ (Name) ______________ (Phone)
3. ______________________ (Name) ______________ (Phone)

OTHER CONSULTANTS

SW: ______________________ (Name) ______________ (Phone)

Other: ______________________ (Name) ______________ (Phone)

DIAGNOSES

1. ______________________ 2. ______________________

3. ______________________

Exacerbating potentials: ______________________________________

I. BIRTH DATA

1. Hospital of Delivery: ______________________
2. History of Prenatal Care: ______________________
3. Gestational Age at Birth: __________ Wgt.: __________

   Problems: ______________________________________
4. Delivery: _____ Vaginal _____ C-Section
5. Condition of Baby at Delivery/Complications

II. CURRENT STATE OF HEALTH

1. Physical
2. Mental
3. Emotional
4. Social
5. Hospitalizations/Surgeries

III. CHILD'S HEALTH CARE NEEDS: (Specify with as much detail as possible)

I. Diet/Feeding Schedule:

2. Activity:

3. Physical Therapy:

4. Psychological Therapy/OT:

5. Educational Therapies:

6. Speech Therapy:

7. Equipment and use including tubes present—source of equipment—who supplies:

8. Medications—name, dose, route, freq., purpose:

9. Teaching Needed:

_____ Nutrition

_____ Growth/dev.

_____ Formula prep and access to formula

_____ Parenting education

_____ Budgeting of financial resources

_____ Home safety

_____ Parenting

_____ Community resources

_____ Utilities

_____ Phone

_____ Housing

_____ Cooking

_____ Water

_____ Respite

_____ Others

10. Referrals already made: ______________________________

11. Referrals needed: ______________________________

_____ Kencrest _____ Other

IV. FAMILY DATA/SUPPORT NETWORK

1. Primary Caretaker of Child

Name: ______________________

Health Status: ______________________

Ed. Issues: ______________________

Age: ________

2. Siblings (Name, Age, Address, Medical Issues, Parents):

_______ no. of Siblings:

3. Other Household Members (Name, Age, Medical Issues):

4. Other Significant Others/Extended Family Members. Are they available to assist with care of child—when?

5. Summary of Household Function—Do people work together? Do they get along, who is in charge, etc.:

6. Evidence of Drug/alcohol Use:

V. HOUSING INFORMATION:

1. Current Residence: _____ permanent _____ temporary

2. Type of Residence: _____ sngle Family _____ apt. _____ shelter

3. Length of Time in Current Residence: _____________

4. Are there Plans for Move? _____ Yes _____ When? _____ No

   New Address: ___________________________________

5. Layout of House: _______ no. of Bedrooms _______ no. of Bathrooms _______ kitchen
   _______ living Area _______ furniture _______ dining Area

   Condition of House: ____

6. Safety issues at House:

   Outlets: _____ 2-prong _____ 3-prong _____ adeq. No.'s _____ inadeq. No.'s

   Smoke Alarms: Yes _____ No _____ no. of alarms: _____

   Stable Railings: Yes _____ No _____

   Adequate Lighting: Yes _____ No _____ Specify: ____

   Emergency No.'s Posted: Yes _____ No _____

   Sanitation: No. of Bathrooms: _______

   A. Is kitchen sanitary: Yes _____ No _____ Specify: ____

   B. Pest Control: Are the following present:

   _____ roaches _____ rats/Mice _____ flies

   C. Plumbing problems ____

Medication storage—specify plan for storage, if refrigeration needed:

Infection control needs surrounding care:

7. Will house need modification/rearrangement for child (specify):

8. Specify space child will have to sleep, play, exercise, etc., and equipment (bed, toys) available:

VI. FINANCIAL DATA

1. Source of income for parent/guardian Name: ______________________________

   _____ DPA Amount $ ________________ _____ SSI Amount $ ________________

   _____ Job Amount $ ________________

   _____ Other: Specify type/amount: ____

   _____ Child Support Amount $ ________________

2. Income Supplements—Program Participation

   _____ WIC _____ Food Stamps $ ________________

   _____ Public housing Rent $ ________________

   _____ Section VIII housing Amount $ ________________

   _____ School lunch _____ School breakfast

3. Expenses—Specify Amount

   _____ Rent $ ________________ _____ Food $ ________________

   _____ Utilities $ ________________ _____ Meds $ ________________

   _____ Trans. $ ________________ _____ Clothing $ ________________

4. HEALTH INSURANCE:

   _____ MA _____ HMA _____ NONE _____ Other: ________________

   _____ NEEDS ASSIST—Specify:

SUMMARY OF CLIENT:

BARRIERS TO HEALTH CARE DELIVERY/PLAN IMPLEMENTATION:

PROBLEM LIST—PRELIMINARY:

Appendix L

Discharge Summary

Insurance Co.: ______________________ ID#: ______________________

Client Name: ______________________ Date of Birth: ______________________

Address: ______________________

Diagnosis: ______________________

Date of First Visit: __________ Date of Last Visit: __________

No. of Visits: RN: ______ LPN: ______ PT: ______ OT: ______ ST: ______ HHA: ______ Other: __________
(type of service)

Date of Discharge: __________

Initiation of Discharge: Physician (give name): ______________________

Physician's Address: ______________________

Agency: __________ Client/Family: __________

Reason for termination of service: ______________________

____

Summary of Progress and Client/Patient Status at Discharge (Physical, Mental, Emotional):

SUBJECTIVE: ______________________

____

____

OBJECTIVE: ______________________

____

ASSESSMENT: ______________________

____

____

GOALS:	ATTAINED	
______________	Yes: ______	No: ______
______________	Yes: ______	No: ______
______________	Yes: ______	No: ______

PLAN
Referrals made and final disposition: ______________________

____

____

Client/Patient notified of discharge: Yes: ______ No: ______ Family notified of discharge: Yes: ______ No: ______

Physician notified of discharge: Yes: ______ No: ______

Signature: ______________________ Date: __________

Appendix M

High-Risk Follow-Up Program Case Management Log

Measureable Outcomes—Plan of Care Goals

Process (date/time of appointments):

Completed:

PLAN	OUTCOME	COMMENTS
BIRTH–2 MONTHS		
At least 1 newborn visit to pediatric provider		
HBV given		
Health insurance for newborn		
Appt. w/caseworker to enroll baby by 2nd wk of age		
Emergency		
Urgent care		
Routine		
Social and financial support		
Food resources		
Adequate maternal foods/fluid		
Adequate newborn resources		
Food stamps		
WIC referral		
Mental health, drug/alcohol counseling		
Newborn wt. gain of 4–6 oz/wk		
Linkage to health care system initiated		
Transp. avail. for medical care appts.		
Insurance provider to initiate newborn enrollment		
WIC appts.		

PLAN	OUTCOME	COMMENTS
ER use and rehosp. prevented		
Parenting problems identified and referral or teaching initiated		
2–4 MONTHS		
Newborn adequately nourished as evidenced by growth and wt. gain		
Developmental milestones reached by age 3 months		
Raise head and chest when lying on stomach		
Stretch legs and kick when lying down		
Bring hands and toys to mouth		
Reach for dangling objects		
Grasp and shake toys like rattles		
Recognize familiar objects and people		
Follow moving objects with eyes		
Watch your facial expression		
Smile and babble		
Enjoy people, including strangers		
Linkages to health care		
Brute. in place		
Pediatric provider appt. for immunizations kept		
At 2 months DPT–polio, HIB		
At 4 mos. DPT–polio, HIB		
Lead level determined		
Referrals previously initiated in place		
EPSDT program		
4–6 MONTHS		
Growth adequate for age		
Developmental milestones reached by age 6 mos.		
Work hard to get objects that are out of reach		
Find partially hidden toys		
Respond to own name and familiar words		
Babble in response to your speech		

PLAN	OUTCOME	COMMENTS
Sit with help		
Roll stomach to back		
Reach for and grab toys		
Pediatric provider appt. for immunizations kept		
At 6 months. DPT–polio, HIB, HBV		
Lead level drawn at 6 mos and result known		
Nutritional support and teaching		
Adequate food available		
Transition from all formula to baby foods started		
Follow-up with community resource linkages to which family previously referred		
6–8 MONTHS		
Growth adequate for age		
Developmental milestones reached		
Any outstanding problems previously listed		
8–10 MONTHS		
Lead level drawn by 9 mos. if first result was >10–14 μg/dl		
Any outstanding problems previously listed		
10–12 MONTHS		
Lead level drawn by 12 mos. if first result was < 10 μg/dl		
Any outstanding problems previously listed		
Discharge Planning		

Appendix **N**

Record Audit Form for Collection of High-Risk Newborn Follow-Up Data

Newborn Name: ______________________ Date of Service: ____________

ADM: ____________ D/C: ____________ No. of visits: ____________

Describe problems in carrying out plan of care: ______________________

____

____

Is it known if client has working phone? Yes _____ No _____

Was newborn difficult to locate at times? If yes, describe: ______________________

____

____

Do there appear to be language barriers: Yes _____ No _____

Do notes reflect dates of newborn's pediatric appointments? Yes _____ No _____

Describe: ____

____

Do notes reflect if newborn attended pediatric appointments? Yes _____ No _____

Do notes reflect illnesses which may have delayed immunizations or gotten infant off traditional schedule?

Yes _____ No _____

Is there a data outcome form retrievable for this newborn? Yes _____ No _____

Describe any insurance changes: ____

Do notes reflect primary care at any other location? Yes _____ No _____

Immunization status:

	Up to date	Not up to date
DPT:	_____	_____
OPY:	_____	_____
HIB:	_____	_____
HBV:	_____	_____
TB:	_____	_____

Appendix O

High-Risk Newborn Follow-Up Program

Chart Review

Name: ________________________________ Date: ________________

Admission date: ________________ Insurance type at admission: ________________

Discharge date: ________________ Insurance type at discharge: ________________

Length of service (wks): ________________ Total no. of visits: ________________

Hospital admission: Yes _____ No _____

Dates and Diagnosis: ____

ER Visit: Yes _____ No _____

Dates and Diagnosis: ____

REASON FOR DISCHARGE:

Not home for Scheduled Visit _______ Newborn Death (home) _______

Refused visit(s) _______ Insurer denied authorization _______

Moved/unable to locate _______ Improved condition/stable _______

Newborn Hospitalized _______ Noncompliant _______

Other: ____

Appendix P

Newborn Quantitative Data

Monthly and quarterly data collection: Disposition of newborn

Referrals

Universal newborn screenings

Maternal/newborn referrals: ________

- No. refused visit: ________
- No. unable to locate: ________
- No. ineligible per ins. co.: ________
- No. misc. (no-show, moved, hosp, foster placement): ________

Total no. not visited of referrals made: ________

Total no. patients seen: ________

- No. newborns: ________
- No. maternal patients: ________
- No. visits: ________
- No. newborn patients: ________
- No. visits: ________

Total no. cases visited and opened for follow-up of risk factors identified at hospital discharge or newborn home visit other than high-risk admission criteria: ________

- No. maternal patients: ________
- No. visits: ________
- No. newborn patients: ________
- No. visits: ________

Total # cases opened for follow-up of high-risk admission criteria

No. newborns remaining in service after 62 days:

- No prenatal care: ________
- Teen, <17 years old: ________
- Substance abuse: ________
- Lack of adequate prenatal care: ________
- Other: ________

Percent of referrals opened for follow-up due to risk and problems (of high-risk admission criteria) identified: ________

Percent of referrals opened for follow-up of high-risk admission criteria and risk level categories: ________

Appendix Q

Newborn Qualitative Data

Total # newborns seen ________

________ Reports of illness or changes in condition by nurse to practitioner

________ Emergency room visits

________ Rehospitalizations

________ Identification of primary care for follow-up

________ Identification of WIC

________ Identification of insurance

________ No. newborns meeting high risk admission criteria

________ No. newborns followed in home care beyond 62 days meeting high risk admission criteria

Appendix R

Outcome Data for Newborns in High-Risk Follow-Up

Patient Name: ______________________________ DOS: ______________

Admission Date: ______________ Pediatric F/U Site: __________________________

Birth Weight: ________

		Appropriate for Age		
Weights:	3 mos	_____ Y	_____ N	_____ NA
	6 mos	_____ Y	_____ N	_____ NA
	9 mos	_____ Y	_____ N	_____ NA
	12 mos	_____ Y	_____ N	_____ NA

Lead screen done at or by age 6 mos.: _____ Y _____ N _____ NA

Lead Level: ____________ Plan for followup (if applicable):

Other important data regarding illness (explain):

Illness: _____ Y _____ N

ER Visit: _____ Y _____ N

Hospitalization: _____ Y _____ N

Referrals to Child Protective Service: _____ Y _____ N

Transfer to another pediatric provider for follow-up:

_____ Y (specify name): ______________________________ N _____

Unable to determine follow-up site: _____ Y _____ N

IMMUNIZATIONS (LIST ALL DATES):

DPT:	_____ Y	_____ N	_____ NA
Oral Polio Vaccine:	_____ Y	_____ N	_____ NA
MMR:	_____ Y	_____ N	_____ NA
HIS:	_____ Y	_____ N	_____ NA
HIBV:	_____ Y	_____ N	_____ NA
TB:	_____ Y	_____ N	_____ NA
Other:	_____ Y	_____ N	_____ NA

Appropriately immunized for age: _____ Y _____ N

Common Abbreviations in Maternal–Child Nursing

ABC	alternative birthing center; airway, breathing, circulation
AC	abdominal circumference
ADA	American Diabetes Association
ADL	activities of daily living
AFP	alpha-fetoprotein
AFV	amniotic fluid volume
AGA	average for gestational age
AIDS	acquired immune deficiency syndrome
AROM	artificial rupture of membranes
BAT	brown adipose tissue (brown fat)
BGS	blood glucose sample
bili	blood bilirubin level
BL	baseline (fetal heart rate baseline)
BMR	basal metabolic rate
BOW	bag of waters
BP	blood pressure
BPD	biparietal diameter; bronchopulmonary dysplasia
BPM	beats per minute
BSE	breast self-examination
BUN	blood urea nitrogen
CC	chest circumference; cord compression; chief complaint
cc	cubic centimeter
CDC	Centers for Disease Control
CF	cystic fibrosis
CHF	congestive heart failure
CID	cytomegalic inclusion disease
CMV	cytomegalovirus
cm	centimeter
CNM	certified nurse-midwife
CNS	central nervous system
CPAP	continuous positive airway pressure
CPD	cephalopelvic disproportion; citrate–phosphate–dextrose
CPR	cardiopulmonary resuscitation
C/S	cesarean section or c-section
DD	developmental disability
DHS	Department of Health Services
dil	dilatation
D&C	dilatation and curettage
DES	diethylstilbestrol

DFMR	daily fetal movement response
DM	diabetes mellitus
DNR	do not resucitate
DOB	date of birth
DRG	diagnostic related groups
DTR	deep tendon reflexes
ECMO	extracorporeal membrane oxygenator
EDC	estimated date or confinement
EFA	essential fatty acid
EFM	electronic fetal monitoring
EFW	estimated fetal weight
EI	early intervention
EPIS	episiotomy
FAD	fetal activity diary
FAS	fetal alcohol syndrome
FBS	fetal blood sample; fasting blood sugar
FBM	fetal breathing movements
FHR	fetal heart rate
FHT	fetal heart tones
FM	fetal movement
FMD	fetal movement diary
FMR	fetal movement record
FPG	fasting plasma glucose
FTT	failure to thrive
G&D	growth and development
GDM	gestational diabetes mellitus
GI	gastrointestinal
GRAV	gravida
GT	gastrostomy tube
GTT	glucose tolerance test
GYN	gynecology
HAL	hyperalimentation
HCG	human chorionic gonadotrophin
HEENT	head, ears, eyes, nose, throat
HIV	human immunodeficiency virus
IDDM	insulin-dependent diabetes mellitus
IGT	impaired glucose tolerance
IL	intralipids
ITP	idiopathis thrombocytopenic purpura
IUFD	intrauterine fetal demise
IUGR	intrauterine growth retardation
IV	intravenous
JCAHO	Joint Commission for the Accreditation of Healthcare Organizations
L/S ratio	lecithin/sphingomyelin ratio
MAP	mean arterial pressure
MCH	maternal–child health
MH	mental health
MR	mental retardation
NG	nasogastric tube
NIDDM	non–insulin-dependent diabetes mellitus
NKA	no know allergies
NPO	nulla per os
NSCT	nipple stimulation challenge test
NST	non-stress test
OB	obstetric

OCT	oxytocin challenge test
OES	oral electrolyte solution
ORS	oral rehydration solution
ORT	oral rehydration therapy
Peds	pediatrids
PIH	pregancy-induced hypertension
PO	per os (by mouth)
PROM	premature rupture of membranes
RBC	red blood cell
RDS	Respiratory distress syndrome
RMA	right mentoanterior
ROA	right occiput anterior
ROM	rupture of membranes
ROP	right occiput posterior
ROP	retinopathy of prematurity
ROT	right occiput transverse
RMP	right mentoposterior
RMT	right mentotransverse
RSA	right sacroanterior
RSP	right sacroposterior
SFD	small for dates
SGA	small for gestational age
SIDS	sudden infant death syndrome
SOAP	subjective data, objective data, analysis, plan
SOB	short of breath
SROM	spontaneous rupture of the membranes
S/S	signs and symptoms
STD	sexually transmitted disease
TORCH	toxoplasmosis, other (viruses) rubella, cytomegalovirus, herpes virus type 2
TPN	total parenteral nutrition
TSS	toxic shock syndrome
U/A	urinalysis
UAC	umbilical artery catheter
UC	uterine contraction
UPI	uteroplacental insufficiency
UTI	urinary tract infection
VBAC	vaginal birth after cesarean
WBC	white blood cell
WIC	supplemental food program for woman, infants, and children
WNL	within normal limits

Glossary

abortion loss of pregnancy before the fetus is viable outside the uterus; miscarriage, or elective termination

abruptio placentae partial or total premature separation of a normally implanted placenta.

acceleration increase in the baseline fetal heart

acme peak; time of greatest intensity (of a uterine contraction)

acrocyanosis cyanosis of the extremities

afterbirth placenta and membranes expelled or "delivered" after the infant; referred to as the third stage of labor

afterbirth pains cramplike pains due to contractions of the uterus after childbirth

albinism a congenital absence of normal skin pigmentation

albuminuria readily detectable amounts of albumin in the urine

amenorrhea suppression or absence of menstruation

amniocentesis removal of amniotic fluid by insertion of needle into the amniotic sac (amniotic fluid is used to assess health and maturity status of fetus)

amnion the inner of the two uterine membranes that form the sac containing the fetus and the amniotic fluid

amniotic fluid the fluid surrounding the fetus in utero

amnionitis infection within the amniotic fluid

amniotomy the artificial rupturing of the amniotic sac

analgesic drug that relieves pain

anencephaly congenital deformity in which the cerebrum, cerebellum, and flat bones of the skull are absent

anesthesia partial or complete loss of sensation with or without loss of consciousness; excess amount of carbon dioxide in the body

anomaly a malformation; an organ or structure

anoxia deficiency of oxygen

antepartum time between conception and the onset of labor

anterior pertaining to the front

Apgar score a scoring system used to evaluate newborns at 1 minute and 5 minutes after delivery. The total score is derived by assessing five signs: heart rate, respiratory effort, muscle tone, reflex irritability, and color

apnea a condition that occurs when respirations cease for more than 20 seconds, with cyanosis

areola darker pigmented skin surrounding the nipple of the breast

Bartholin's glands	two small mucus glands on each side of the vaginal orifice that secrete small amounts of mucus during intercourse
bilirubin	orange or yellowish pigment in bile; a breakdown product of red blood cells that is carried by the blood to the liver, where it is excreted in the bile and in the stools.
brown adipose tissue	fat deposits in neonates that provide greater heat protection
caudal block	regional anesthesia used in childbirth, given through the spinal canal
cephalhematoma	subcutaneous swelling found on the head of an infant several days after delivery
cephalic	referring to the head
cervical dilation	the cervical os and the cervical canal widen from less than 1 centimeter to approximately 10 centimeters
chloasma	brownish pigmentation over the bridge of the nose
chorion	one of the two uterine membranes closest to the intrauterine wall
Leopold's maneuvers	series of four maneuvers designed to allow the examiner to determine fetal presentation and position
mastitis	inflammation of the breast
neonatal mortality rate	number of deaths of infants in the first 28 days of life per 1,000 live births
neonate	infant from birth through the first 28 days of life
neonatology	the specialty that focuses on the management of high-risk conditions of the newborn
omphalitis	infection of the umbilicus
omphalocele	congential herniation of abdominal contents into the base of the umbilicus
outlet dystocia	inadequate pelvic size, causing the fetal head to be pushed backward toward the coccyx, making delivery of head difficult
ovum	female reproductive cell; egg
oxygen toxicity	serious, sometimes irreversible damage to pulmonary capillary endothelium associated with excessive levels of oxygen therapy
oxytocics	drugs that stimulate uterine contractions
oxytocin	hormone normally produced by the posterior pituitary, responsible for stimulation of uterine contractions and the release of milk into the lactiferous ducts
oxytocin challenge test (OCT)	also called the contraction stress test (CCST), the test evaluates the circulatory and respiratory status of the fetoplacental unit
palpation	use of fingers or hands to manually perform assessment
perforation of the uterus	a hole made in the uterus
perineum	the area of tissue between the anus and vagina in the female
periodic breathing	sporadic episodes of apnea, not associated with cyanosis, lasting about 10 seconds
persistent pulmonary hypertension	a neonatal syndrome secondary to pulmonary hypertension; seen in preterm but more frequently in full-term and postmature infants

phenylketonuria (PKU)	a recessive hereditary metabolic error that causes the buildup of phenylalanine, leading to mental retardation, brain damage, light pigmentation and other growth deformities. It is treated with a low-phenylalanine diet
phlebitis	inflammation of a vein
phototherapy	treatment of newborn jaundice by exposure to natural or special artificial light
physiologic jaundice	harmless condition caused by the normal reduction of red blood cells, occurs usually between the second and fifth day after birth, peaking on the fifth to seventh day, and disappearing between the seventh and tenth day.
placenta previa	improper implantation of the placenta on the lower uterine segment. Classification of type is based on closeness to the cervical os: total—completely covers the os; partial—covers a portion of the os; marginal—in close proximity to the os
preterm infant	any infant born before 37 weeks' gestation
preterm labor	labor beginning before the 37th week of gestation
primipara	a woman who has given birth to her first child
postmature infant	a newborn that is overly developed or that is more than 42 weeks' gestation
postnatal	occurring after birth
precipitous delivery	unduly rapid progression of labor
preeclampsia	toxemia of pregnancy; characterized by hypertension, albuminuria, and edema
pregnancy-induced hypertension (PIH)	a hypertensive disorder including preeclampsia and identified by the three cardinal signs: hypertension, edema, and proteinuria
prolapsed cord	umbilical cord that becomes compressed in the vagina before the fetus is delivered, resulting in emergency situation for the fetus
prolonged labor	labor lasting more than 24 hours
puerperium	the period after completion of the third stage of labor until involution of the uterus is complete at about 6 weeks
quickening	the first fetal movements felt by the pregnant woman, usually between 16 and 18 weeks' gestation
rales	an abnormal respiratory sound caused by air passing through fluid in the alveoli and bronchioles
regional anesthesia	injection of local anesthetic
rhonchi	coarse, abnormal auscultatory sounds
saddle block anesthesia	sensory and motor anesthesia of the buttocks, perineum, and inner aspects of the thighs, produced by spinal or intrathecal injection
show	a pinkish mucous discharge from the vagina that may occur a few hours to a few days before the onset of labor
spina bifida occulta	a defect in the vertebrae of the spinal column without protrusion of neural components
subinvolution	failure of a part to return to its normal size
surfactant	a surface-active mixture of secreted lipoproteins caused by *Candida albicans*, in the alveoli and air passages; it reduces surface tension of pulmonary fluids and contributes to the elasticity of lung tissue
tachycardia	abnormally rapid heart rate

tachypnea	excessively rapid respirations
term infant	a liveborn infant at 38 to 42 weeks' gestation
thromboembolus	thrombotic material or clot within the vein
tocodynamometer	external device that can be used to estimate uterine contraction pressures during labor
umbilical cord	the structure connecting the placenta to the umbilicus of the fetus through which the fetus receives nutrition and eliminates wastes
urinary meatus	external opening of the urethra
uterus	the hollow muscular organ in which the fertilized egg is implanted and in which the developing fetus is nourished until birth
vagina	the musculomembranous tube located between the external genitals and the uterus
varicose veins	permanently distended veins
vasectomy	surgical removal of a portion of the vas deferens

Index

Note: Page numbers followed by *t* indicate tables.